PRAISE FOR

THE LAST DOCTOR

National Bestseller

Finalist for the 2022 Writers' Trust
Balsillie Prize for Public Policy

A *Hill Times* 2022 Best Book of the Year

"A remarkable book. . . . Extremely well-written, touching, full of love and nuance. Some humour, too, because both life and death are full of it. It is a must-read for anyone who wishes to understand the issue better." —*Ottawa Citizen*

"[This] wise, humane, and yes, humorous, account of Marmoreo's end-of-life practice features a cast of memorable, vividly drawn characters. . . . Deftly weaving memoir and the changing complexities of Canadian law, the book centres on Marmoreo's self-portrait—a woman who is not afraid to admit she was wrong, who can change her mind, and whose work with the dying forces her to reconsider life, death, dignity, loneliness, and the Canadian medical system."
—Katherine Ashenburg, author of *The Mourner's Dance: What We Do When People Die* and *Her Turn*

"[A] compassionate and courageous memoir of [Marmoreo's] pioneering work. . . . The book you must read before talking about your end of life wishes with your loved ones and your legal and medical advisors." —Sandra Martin, author of *A Good Death: Making the Most of Our Final Choices*

"*The Last Doctor* is a majestic book about the power of kindness and the language of love. It will change forever how you think about medically assisted dying. Your end-of-life self will love, honour, and cherish Dr. Jean's insights." —Dr. Joe MacInnis, author of *Deep Leadership*

"A reminder of the fragility of life [as well as] the inside and honest story of a medical doctor tackling her own fragility and personal history. . . . This book offers the hope that we all need." —Dr. Roberta Bondar, astronaut, scientist, physician, writer, photographer

"Dr. Marmoreo's commitment, intelligence, fierceness, frustration, humour, and, most importantly, compassion come through on every page. If you want to understand the sometimes messy sometimes tidy, sometimes simple sometimes complex, and always profound world of medical assistance in dying—read this book." —Jocelyn Downie, CM, FRSC, FCAHS, SJD, Professor in the Faculties of Law and Medicine, Dalhousie University

THE LAST DOCTOR

THE
LAST
DOCTOR

Lessons in Living from
the Front Lines of
Medical Assistance in Dying

DR. JEAN MARMOREO
and JOHANNA SCHNELLER

PENGUIN

an imprint of Penguin Canada,
a division of Penguin Random House Canada Limited

First published in Viking hardcover by Penguin Canada, 2022
Published in this edition, 2024

1 2 3 4 5 6 7 8 9 10

LIBRARY AND ARCHIVES CANADA CATALOGUING IN PUBLICATION

Title: The last doctor : lessons in living from the front lines of medical
assistance in dying / Dr. Jean Marmoreo and Johanna Schneller.
Names: Marmoreo, Jean, author. | Schneller, Johanna, author.
Identifiers: Canadiana 20230195563 | ISBN 9780735248397 (softcover)
Subjects: LCSH: Marmoreo, Jean—Anecdotes. | LCSH: Assisted suicide—Canada. |
LCSH: Assisted suicide—Canada—Anecdotes.
Classification: LCC R726 .M37 2024 | DDC 616.02/9—dc23

Book design by Emma Dolan
Cover design and art by Emma Dolan
Typeset by Terra Page

Printed in the United States of America

www.penguinrandomhouse.ca

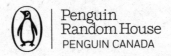

Penguin
Random House
PENGUIN CANADA

For Yolanda Martins,
whose generosity and grace in her quest for a dignified
death prompted an inner journey, and this book.

WILD GEESE

You do not have to be good.
You do not have to walk on your knees
for a hundred miles through the desert, repenting.
You only have to let the soft animal of your body
    love what it loves.
Tell me about despair, yours, and I will tell you mine.
Meanwhile the world goes on.
Meanwhile the sun and the clear pebbles of the rain
are moving across the landscapes,
over the prairies and the deep trees,
the mountains and the rivers.
Meanwhile the wild geese, high in the clean blue air,
are heading home again.
Whoever you are, no matter how lonely,
the world offers itself to your imagination,
calls to you like the wild geese, harsh and exciting –
over and over announcing your place
in the family of things.

—Mary Oliver

Contents

Yolanda, Part One

I was supposed to administer the drugs that would end Yolanda Martins's life at ten a.m. There was only one problem: I needed a nurse to insert the intravenous lines, and the nurse hadn't arrived.

The mood in the house had already gone up and down more times than an elevator. About a dozen of Yolanda's friends and family—a vivacious, urbane bunch—were gathered in this meticulously renovated Victorian in Toronto's Annex neighbourhood, owned by Yolanda's friend Patty, to send her off. Someone had hung up strings of white fairy lights. Someone had made coffee; someone else had opened tequila and champagne, and it seemed like every glass in the kitchen was in use. Bunches of flowers and boxes of tissues sat on the large square kitchen island, and on every other surface, too. Yolanda, who had a sly sense of humour, had made an upbeat "death playlist," and she and her loved ones had spent the last hour chatting, crying, dancing, laughing, and belting out the lyrics to "Forever Young" and "Karma Chameleon." But as ten a.m. came and went, people's eyes started flicking to me.

By this July day in 2018, almost eighteen months since I'd first helped a person to die, I'd experienced repeatedly the tremendous good in it. The relief on patients' faces when they give their final consent. The mournful yet joyful gatherings, like this one for Yolanda, to witness loved ones dying by their own rules, often in their own beds. The family members who hugged me afterward, who sat down close beside me to tell me stories about the person to whom they'd just bade farewell. That's when I would cry. I almost always cry.

I first met Yolanda back in November 2017. She was one of the certain ones. She was only forty-five, but she'd been sick with a rare lung disease for thirty years. Yet somehow she'd lived a big life: she was a scientific researcher at Harvard; she'd jumped out of planes and dived deep to coral reefs. She had a forceful personality. Her friends jokingly called her the Boss. They loved saying that what Yolanda wanted, Yolanda got. But in the last two years, that big life had narrowed—it began to consist mainly of medicines, paperwork, pain. She had no money, no boyfriend; her energy was gone, her concentration dwindling. She had to move back to her parents' house in Whitby, a town about an hour east of Toronto, with short stays here at Patty's. Yolanda was becoming less and less herself. She was ready to go.

Now that day had arrived. Yolanda had dressed for it in a watery-blue silk kimono, a striped shirt, leggings, and little velvet slippers. She also wore a clear plastic oxygen tube slung around her neck and tucked into her nostrils. The cord on the oxygen tank was long enough that she could move throughout the open-concept first floor, from living room to dining area to kitchen, playing hostess at her own death cocktail party. Time ticked by. It's not that everyone wanted me to begin Yolanda's end, but they'd steeled themselves for a certain hour. The extra minutes were welcome but also awkward.

My eyes, meanwhile, kept flicking to the door. I had discreetly phoned my office. We use a community home care service, with nurses very skilled at inserting IV lines in frail, elderly patients. The agency had acknowledged my request. So where was the nurse? Feeling some urgency now, I called my go-to person, Yuri. He has a preternatural serenity that makes you feel anything is doable. He was in a meeting, but he agreed to jump in his car and come right away.

At 10:20, I made an announcement. "We try to plan this day as carefully as possible, but sometimes things happen," I said. I'm always direct. I've learned it's what people want.

By the time they've reached this point—this terminus—they don't need euphemisms. They know where they are and why.

"The nurse who was to start the IV hasn't come," I explained. "But there is a nurse on the way now. Twenty minutes or so."

A beat of silence, then the chatting and music resumed. Yolanda's brother sprinted up the street to the liquor store— it opened at ten a.m., a weird silver lining—and came back with more champagne. Someone turned up the music.

There was one more issue, but I didn't mention it, and neither did Yolanda. Most medical assistance in dying (MAiD) provisions aren't time-sensitive. The end will arrive; a few minutes here or there won't change that. But Yolanda's came with a deadline. When she knew—really, fully knew— that she was going to die, she was adamant that it not be in vain. She would donate her lungs, etched as they were with the mysterious runes of her disease, to the pathologists at Toronto General Hospital. They'd booked an operating room for one p.m. to remove them. I'd booked a funeral home to transport her body from Patty's house to the hospital and then back to the funeral home. I would not—could not—fail her in this. I'd promised her that I'd get this done.

I was determined to remain calm. But Yolanda—she didn't have to fake it. She was there, in the zone, in the certainty. This moment had been coming for her for most of her young life. Instead of shrinking from it, she was pulling it close. I kept thinking of what she'd said to me in the spring, after her formal request for spiritual guidance had fallen through one of the gaping cracks in the system I'd referred her to: she was so tired of carrying her burden all alone.

We had tried. But while all kinds of support were in place for in-hospital patients, there wasn't an outreach person for people in Yolanda's situation, living with her fatal disease at home. The hospital team, who'd tried to connect her with a spiritual advisor, was apologetic. I was apologetic.

But after the advisor failed to materialize, Yolanda had come up with a new plan. "You will tell my story," she said to me. It was not a request.

So here we go.

CHAPTER ONE

The Beginning

February 6, 2015. A bleary day. At seven a.m., I was on a treadmill, finishing my pre-office workout at a downtown gym. The TV screens above me were tuned to the news—ordinary stuff, traffic, weather. I was half-watching, my overly busy schedule running through my overly busy brain.

Then game-changing words scrolled across the screen. After a long battle, the Supreme Court of Canada had ruled in a landmark case, *Carter v. Canada*. The decision was unanimous, nine to zero: prohibiting an individual who had a serious illness or disease from requesting an assisted death was counter to the Canadian Charter of Rights and Freedoms, specifically the rights to life, liberty, and security of the person. The court recognized that sections of the Criminal Code prohibiting physicians from assisting such patients were unconstitutional. It gave governments in each province and territory one year to frame the legislative changes required to reflect the new law.

In other words, in one year, Canadians who previously had to face the grimmest of choices—suffer in agony or seek an illegal back door to death—would be allowed to request and receive a humane, reliable, legal end.

I stepped off the treadmill and stared at the screen, panting. I was stunned in the first breath, thrilled in the next, and resolute by the third: this would be my next job—and my last. I had long believed in assisted death, but I never thought it would happen in my lifetime. Now I could close out my forty-five-year career as a physician by helping people end their lives their way.

Looking back on that time, I see a certain bravura on my part. This is the right thing to do! I am the right person to do it! After nearly five decades in family practice in Toronto, I had experienced the value of a long, thorough, personal relationship between a patient and their family doctor. My ideal was cradle-to-grave care: to begin with a patient in young adulthood and stay with them until the end. My younger patients often said, "You cannot retire before I die!" and my response was always, "I'll be dead before you, never fear."

But there were many patients for whom I could not provide the end-of-life care they sought. The gravely ill and those facing dementia didn't want me to prolong their lives. They wanted me to ease them out. They didn't want to linger in terrible pain, dependent on others for their most basic personal care. They didn't want to deteriorate until they no longer recognized their own children. Too many of these patients had disappeared from my care, abruptly. Knowing them so intimately, I understood why: they were taking matters into their own hands. They couldn't tell me, because I'd be criminally liable if there was any inkling that I had helped them.

All of my patients expected me to advocate for them, to secure their best possible care. For most, an assisted death was low on their list of considerations. Only a small percentage would ever request it, I knew. But now that that service was becoming legal, I wanted to provide it.

Over the years, I'd witnessed individual health care becoming increasingly fractured—farmed out to specialty clinics, oncologists, cancer wards, palliative teams. People want specialists, and I understand that. But in those clinics, the condition is the primary focus, not always the person. I had become under-involved in providing that natural extension of care—the end-of-life piece—for seriously ill people whom I knew literally inside out. I also had a number of older patients who'd been with me for decades; as they moved into long-term care facilities, they faced increasing difficulties getting to my clinic.

On top of that, when a patient experiences more and more emergency room visits and subsequent hospitalizations, our system of care assigns them to chronic care units, where a medical director takes over. Every occurrence—from a fall to confusion, from a failing heart to shortness of breath—binds my patients more firmly to hospitals or ER physicians, rather than to me. I realized that if I were to take on medical assistance to die, I'd better be ready to take on the whole package of end-of-life care.

But how would I learn to do this? Helping someone to die might no longer be a criminal act, but what did that mean in practice? There were no courses I could take. I knew that MAiD involved a lot of drugs—to put a person to sleep, to paralyze their lungs, to stop their hearts—but they certainly weren't drugs I'd ever worked with in family practice.

As well, I knew that MAiD involved a lot of decisions. I needed to reframe how I talked to patients about their deaths, in order to understand why they would request to be assessed for assisted death. I would have to arm myself with information, to be able to engage in the debate that was already raging between palliative care advocates and MAiD advocates.

Palliative care is specialized medical care for a patient who is living with an incurable, life-threatening illness. Palliative care doctors focus on a patient's quality of life and management of their symptoms. Not only do they help patients understand their options and alternatives, they also tend to the care for patient and family alike. They secure the supports required to ensure a level of comfort. Palliative care often segues into hospice care, where doctors switch from supporting patients in treatment to easing them gently into death. Some palliative care advocates believe that if a patient's pain is under control and their other needs are managed, they have no reason to ask for an assisted death. But assisted death advocates disagree—because we see so many reasons for MAiD beyond pain.

Until MAiD became legal, that debate had been relegated to the hospital teams attached to cancer clinics, where death, though difficult, is a predictable, step-by-step process. (For example, when your palliative performance scale, or PPS, is x, you have x many weeks left.) Historically, end-of-life-care conversations weren't even given a thought in the cardiac (heart) or nephrology (kidney) clinics. We health care providers needed to have long and frank discussions: what does "quality of life" mean when it means something different for everyone?

As the Supreme Court had decreed, the new MAiD law wouldn't come into effect until June 2016, to give the provinces and territories, which are responsible for implementing health care, a chance to apply it in their own jurisdictions. So I resolved to take that time to create my own year-long program of independent learning.

Today, graduates in family practice can take a nine-month specialty program in palliative care. But that wasn't available when earlier generations of family doctors (like me) began our practices, and I didn't have the time to take it—I still had a thriving practice to run. Instead, I decided to trade the two days a week I spent doing obstetrical care for two days of palliative care, shadowing the best practitioners I could find. I would closely observe all kinds of end-of-life quandaries to help me eventually practise MAiD. Furthermore, I would experience patient care from three distinct points of view: in-hospital palliative care, community care in both urban and in rural areas, and hospice care. I would drop in to each of these areas, where doctors and nurses would welcome me with open arms and teach me all I needed to know.

Or so I thought.

For the first part of my independent learning plan—in-hospital palliative care—I turned to Dr. Jeff Myers, who was at the time the head of the palliative unit at Sunnybrook Health Sciences Centre as well as head of the Division of Palliative Care at the University of Toronto. Fit, bearded, and younger than I expected for a person of his expertise, he's unparalleled in his inquisitiveness and undaunted by challenge. Jeff (as I soon came to call him) has a commanding presence. But he also has a familiar and direct approach that put me immediately at ease. I'd say he's an energetic guy, but that's an understatement. I'm pretty speedy myself, yet I literally had to run to keep up with him as he traversed the sprawling hospital from floor to floor. He never took elevators, only the stairs. Whenever I was shadowing him, I'd hope for clear weather, because we were forever dashing between buildings.

When I first approached him about teaching me, he was skeptical. "All family doctors do palliative care," he said.

"That's not my experience," I replied, rhyming off the steps that moved my patients away from me as their diseases or conditions worsened—to specialists, to hospitals, to palliative and hospice care—by which point I was no longer their doctor. The times I had been present at the end of a patient's life, my care had consisted of sitting by their bedsides, keeping vigil, supporting their families, being a witness. It had been passive. I sometimes felt ineffectual. That was something I wanted to change. An hour later, Jeff and I were still talking.

Instead of focusing on MAiD, Jeff wanted Canada to direct its health care resources into better and more palliative care. He could see that palliative care physicians were becoming overwhelmed by our aging population, especially in major cities. He was looking for solutions, and I was keen to offer them. For example, I spitballed, what if MAiD and palliative physicians teamed up to do end-of-life consulting and care—that would ease the burden, wouldn't it? Of course, in practice, that would mean I'd be signing on to do home visits and be available around the clock, and it had been a long time since I'd been on call 24/7. But I'm very good at setting problems aside to think about at some later time. I much prefer getting revved up with ideas.

Jeff had begun his palliative care practice on the West Coast, in the early days of HIV/AIDS deaths. He had learned everything he knew about palliation from looking after people who were dying in droves, many from diseases so rare we doctors hadn't seen them outside textbooks.

As he detailed some of his early experiences with HIV, I flashed back to mine: a gay patient, a flight attendant who did the San Francisco–New York run, sitting in my office in 1979, telling me about an unusual skin cancer that was popping up in the gay community. That was Kaposi sarcoma, and it turned out to be a harbinger of AIDS. That same year, the first *New England Journal of Medicine* article outlining an unusual acceleration of this specific skin disorder was published. Once HIV has gained access, a body can't mount an immune response to ward off specific diseases. Kaposi sarcoma was one, and though readily evidenced in skin lesions, it's really the lining of the blood vessels supplying the skin that is damaged. Other organs—lungs, intestines, and stomach—are equally targeted, with devastating effects.

My flight attendant fell ill himself. Soon, I was seeing HIV everywhere, not only in the gay community but in patients who had had blood transfusions. Jeff had been a groundbreaker in caring for people who were dying with ghastly diseases at a frightful rate in an unknown landscape. These patients were ostracized, isolated, damned by many, supported by few. Jeff and I had compassion in common, and I think that sealed our connection. He became my champion in my plan.

Jeff's goals for me went much further than I'd dreamed, and he challenged me in more ways than I'd expected. I thought observation. He said, "Participation." I thought dabbling. He said, "Immersion and expansion." I had sketched out my course, but he made it concrete. He sent me to a community hospital far from the academic setting, where all palliative care was done by family doctors. He also set me up with the best model of hospice care he knew. (I'll get more into those later.)

First, I tagged along after him on his home turf: the metastatic breast cancer clinic at Sunnybrook. I must have looked like his pull-toy, scooting after him down to the ER, and in and out of clinics. We'd race through hospital buildings to provide just-in-time crisis care. We'd do an emergency consultation in a hospital bay, then sprint to a clinic to oversee an urgent need to hydrate a patient, then find ourselves in an impromptu hallway consultation with unprepared family members who were at that moment realizing that death was near for their loved one.

Jeff also thought big picture: he saw problems and found solutions. For example, he had connected the metastatic breast cancer clinic at his hospital with his palliative care service, to smooth out care for patients as their disease advanced. (That they weren't already linked was a typical oversight; that he made it happen confirmed that he was the right teacher for me.) He was on site to handle crises and to be an ear for physicians as they managed sudden or difficult issues with these women. The nurse-managers would spot patients whose symptoms were accelerating, and Jeff or I would step in. The only time he took me to task was when I spent too long, in his estimation, with any one patient. Cancer patients' needs were always pressing, he said. Get quicker! Run!

My plan for three months of twice-weekly sessions with Jeff stretched to six. Cases were complex, and there was so much to learn. By definition, metastatic breast cancer involved many body systems. What were the options for treatment? New approaches and late-phase trials were becoming available almost weekly—did patients meet the criteria? My role was to review symptoms and prescribe specific remedies. But that could be head-spinning: Would prescribing an anti-inflammatory, such as Celebrex, work better for bone pain than an opiate? How long after radiating a metastatic shoulder bone could the patient expect relief? Jeff's goal was simple: to gain a patient more time. Isn't that what everyone wants?

End-of-life issues, I quickly learned, are whole-life issues. Everything is on the table, and everything needs to be decided stat. I was often left dizzy and insecure. My office practice had little of this intense urgency. I admitted to Jeff that I hadn't dealt with the intricacies of this many drugs and dosing schedules in years. As I sat in those clinics, I was forever fearful that I would slip up—make the wrong calculation for increasing the dose of narcotics to relieve pain, or forget the correct brain pathway that relieved nausea as well as pain. Being up to my neck in the world of narcotics and their contraindications was new to me, so I carried a pocket-sized cheat card for rapid reference. (We all did.) But I didn't want to be whipping it out all the time, like some amateur. These women needed my certainty and confidence. The palliative care I'd done until then had never been this active.

As the countdown to the implementation of the law in 2016 continued, hospitals across Canada scrambled to set up policies for assisted death that would meet their own ethics and procedural guidelines. The exceptions were those hospitals that refused to consider it at all, usually for religious reasons. Thankfully, my home base, Women's College Hospital in downtown Toronto, was fully on board.

Already too busy, I just got busier: I volunteered to be a part of a group of twenty-odd Women's College personnel—drawn from nursing and medical staff, the pharmacy, and the departments of anaesthesia, ethics, and social work—that drafted the hospital's MAiD policies. I supplied the group with copies of the policies that had already been created at Mount Sinai, also in downtown Toronto, and at the Ottawa Civic Hospital. Why reinvent the same policy in every institution? That was a waste of time. We needed to be able to trust—and use—the hard work already done by other like-minded professionals.

I was keen to ensure that Women's College designated a few rooms where family doctors could provide assisted death for patients who couldn't die in their homes. Population polls were consistently reporting that over 70 percent of people wanted to die in their own beds, yet the majority of deaths occurred in hospital. I was a vocal champion for making MAiD as personal as possible, and I was heartened by the support I received in those monthly meetings—even as I gasped at the committee's need to justify this service financially in the hospital's business plan.

By June 2016, when MAiD became legal in Canada, I had moved on to phase two of my self-learning program: out-of-hospital palliative care. Sandy Buchman and David Kendal, two experts who were providing community in-home care out of the Temmy Latner Centre for Palliative Care at Mount Sinai Hospital, agreed to haul me about with them as they saw patients throughout Toronto's downtown core. With them, I would soon participate in my first assisted death.

Dr. Sandy Buchman is a warm grandfatherly type, hard-working with a compassionate manner. Dr. David Kendal, stately, senatorial, and semiretired at that time, was still doing community palliative outreach a few days per week. Like me, he spent more time listening to family members than he did concocting medications.

Their work with patients in their homes—wherever those homes may be, in houses, apartments, retirement residences, or long-term care facilities—was similar to what they'd do in a hospital. Additionally, they paid close attention to the needs of caregivers. Whether they're paid professionals, family members, or friends, caregivers are on call every minute, and they needed our help and timely support, too.

Again, I had so much to learn. The end-of-life programs on offer in long-term care facilities were not unkind, but they often smacked of warehousing. In one such place, we screened a patient who'd just moved in. Leaning against all four walls of his single room were stacks of paintings—which turned out to be his collection of exquisite Inuit art. I never had enough time, beyond my limited purpose, to ask the more human questions: who he was, where his life had taken him, and why no one was there to advocate for him.

Down the hall, we assessed a patient with advanced Alzheimer's who had stopped eating and fallen unconscious, for no discernible reason, really. Dr. David (as we all called him) had a kind but frank conversation with the patient's adult daughter about her end-of-life goals for her dad. I watched her face slacken, almost melt, as he spoke. It was hitting her then, in that minute, that her dad would die in this place, and soon. As David calmly suggested there be no feeding tubes, no transfer to hospital, no resuscitation, she wept. But in the end, she agreed with him.

David also advised the staff to lock her father's door, so other patients couldn't wander in. The notion of being bolted in, unresponsive, alone—suddenly, I found myself staggered. Waiting for the elevator, as I watched a first car go by packed with patients, then a second, I was seized with claustrophobia. I nodded toward the stairs—toward escape. David gently shook his head. "This floor is locked," he reminded me, "and we aren't staff." He didn't have to add that my panic was inappropriate. We waited; the elevator came. Still, I was never so glad to breathe outside air.

Permit me an aside: three days later, that patient woke up and started eating. Again, for no apparent reason. Years later, the vast majority of first-wave COVID-19 deaths in Toronto occurred in long-term care facilities. His was one of them.

In an average day, my two guides and I managed four to six calls, at private homes and in facilities. I was often grateful for my first career as a visiting community nurse. I'd worked in the grittier neighbourhoods of Hamilton, where I'd learned to expect the unexpected when I entered a patient's home.

To save time, I'd assess the patient while Sandy or David talked to the family member. The doer in me frequently rose up against my role as an observer. One morning in a private home, I walked into a bedroom to find the patient moaning, semiconscious, and incontinent, while her support workers stood by, apparently helpless. When I said, "Help me clean her," it wasn't exactly a bark, but it had the same effect. As we changed the patient, I assessed her level of consciousness, her response to pain. Sandy was in the living room, deep in conversation with her husband. I caught his eye and mouthed, "She's in severe distress." He took one look and headed out the door to get medication. I stayed with the caregivers, trying to ease their anxiety, assuring them they hadn't done anything wrong.

Sandy was back in twenty minutes, with an injection of morphine prepared and five more standing by, along with instructions for the husband about how to provide his wife relief. Sandy and I didn't say it, but we both knew she'd be dead within hours.

During those weeks, I was also getting a valuable view of how the nursing arm of an outreach palliative team worked. Early one morning I went to the home of Emily O'Connell, the palliative care intake coordinator for Toronto's downtown LHIN, one of the local health integrated networks, now called Home and Community Care Support Services, servicing the greater Toronto region. Every palliative nurse in the city begins their day with a phone hub, a group conversation with the overnight on-call palliative doctor, oncoming nurses, and the coordinator. In twenty to thirty tightly packed minutes, they share vital information about every patient on their list: the overnight calls, pending issues, potential problems. I was impressed with this level of outreach and on-target access that each nurse had at their fingertips as they started their day. Comprehensive, efficient, effective transfer of information and care from and in the field. Full marks!

After that day's call, we headed off on Emily's own round of patient intake. We talked to families about what services and equipment their loved ones would need. We talked about the kind of human help they'd benefit from, both public and private. And, of course, we talked about the expense.

What I saw with Emily I had seen before, both when I was a visiting nurse in Hamilton and when I was doing house calls in my early days as a family doctor in Toronto. The vast majority of the burden of care for a chronically ill patient falls to a family member, most often a mother, partner, or daughter. They toil behind closed doors, through sleepless nights and seemingly endless days, the only bulwark between those they care for and disaster. The demands on them are absolute; the self-sacrifice, incalculable.

The cost to hire professionals to provide that level of service is astronomical. Provincial health insurance may—*may*—cover two to three hours per day, and that's considered a good quality of care. Even private insurance rarely covers the cost of round-the-clock attention. Truly complete end-of-life care at home simply isn't possible for anyone but the wealthy, unless a family member or friend is part of the plan.

The deluge of information stunned many families who were often still in shock that palliative care was now necessary for their family member. Emily would masterfully ease them into their new reality. For me, her example was a godsend. She gave me the practical tools I needed—facts about hospital beds, varieties of extra help, the basics of making a plan of care, all the essentials and options needed to guide people. And soon, MAiD would be added as one more possibility.

Becoming familiar with how home care in Toronto was structured allowed me to connect more directly with different care coordinators in other LHINs after MAiD came into effect. I'd find myself standing next to a nurse on a streetcar, and we'd get to talking about her patients; soon we'd be deep in a personal conversation about what she should do if MAiD ran counter to her beliefs. So many patients who ask for MAiD need nursing care first and foremost, and no one knows that better than the people in the front lines, the caregivers, the family supporters. They see the declines and disasters unfolding first, and I'm grateful that my time with Emily reminded me of that.

This was underscored for me later, after I'd been providing MAiD for some months. I was assessing a woman with advanced cancer, who lived alone. During my assessment, she suddenly needed the toilet, and she couldn't get there without my assistance. Then she was stuck there until I helped her back. A friend who'd been visiting weekly had gotten her this far, but she had left the city.

I couldn't just assess this woman and leave her to fend for herself, so I phoned the nursing care coordinator. When could a nurse come by? Earliest, tomorrow. Could we get her into hospice? Earliest, two weeks. Had no one put a palliative care team in place? Well, until now, the friend had been handling things.

I boiled over with frustration. This wasn't my job. The late-life medical care system had failed this woman, as so often happens. Why should good end-of-life care be a matter of pure luck? Why did some people get proper, tender send-offs, and others were left alone in misery? MAiD proponents and palliative care proponents are often set in opposition to one another, as if they are two competing sides, either/or. But my year of self-education was showing me they are both part of the same stream. Palliative care and assisted dying had to work together, to offer patients the best of care with the broadest of options.

Was the woman I was assessing requesting MAiD only because other care was unavailable? If so, could I approve her request in good conscience? This should have been resolved weeks, if not months, before she'd reached this desperate point. MAiD is a new option, I reminded myself, but it isn't meant to be the last best one because there isn't any other. Things will get better. Surely, we have to get better in helping the misplaced and left-behind people in this world.

I imagined that when I started to provide MAiD, I'd be the harpist who accompanied those who were fully ready to die. But I was learning that I also would be the bullhorn who called in help, so that some could keep living.

In July 2016, the second month after MAiD went into effect, one of Sandy Buchman's patients requested it. Here we go, I thought, steeling myself. Dr. Buchman brought in a colleague, Dr. Narges Khoshnood (now Dr. Hashemi), a lively person who had already done one MAiD provision and seemed at ease with the process. ("Doing a provision," "providing for a patient"—those were the exceedingly polite terms Canadian doctors and lawmakers had settled on for assisted death. The vocabulary in many other countries that allow medical assistance in dying is more direct. In the Netherlands, for example, doctors say, "I killed a patient yesterday.")

I met Dr. Buchman and Dr. Hashemi at the apartment of the patient, a brisk go-getter I'll call Ted. Ted had four witnesses present. Later, I learned they were business associates, not close friends or family members. That explained a lot, because at the time, I was struck by the lack of emotion in Ted's bedroom. In fact, Ted's bed was just a mattress on the floor, because his condo was already being emptied. I'm sure it was efficient. To me, it felt achingly cold.

This was one of Sandy Buchman's first provisions, and he was grateful for our assistance. I was grateful to be an observer. My job was to record on a one-page procedural form the sequence of drugs and the times they were delivered. Mount Sinai also had a nine-part legal consent form, the key component of which was this: the patient must consent in the moment.

Sandy sat on the floor beside Ted's bed and read out each of the statements on the consent form. Ted had a serious illness, disease, or disability. Ted was in an advanced stage of that condition, resulting in an irreversible decline in capability. It was causing Ted grievous and irremediable suffering. Ted had been advised of alternative means to relieve his suffering and had declined. Ted knew the procedure would result in his death. Ted was not being coerced.

By this point Ted was one more thing: irritated. He immediately assented and signed. (Verbal assent is enough, but some patients and doctors like a signature, too, if possible.)

We doctors withdrew to the small kitchen area. I looked at the ten or so bottles and syringes lined up on the counter. What an array! I watched Dr. Hashemi draw the medications into the syringes with practised efficiency. We returned to the bedroom, and Buchman asked Ted one last time, "Do you wish me to proceed?"

Ted responded with an explosion of expletives. But yes.

As for me? I went straight into procedural mode. I had long ago trained myself to do this, and I've been doing it my entire professional life: I shut out everything except what I must do in that moment. I did not think, Shit, for forty-five years I've dedicated myself to keeping my patients alive, and now one is about to die and I am helping him. I thought, This is the time of delivery for drug A. This is the time of delivery for drug B. My job was to record, and I was focused on recording. When I think about it, I'm amazed at what I can shut out. But I don't think about it much.

The first drug, midazolam, put Ted to sleep in seconds. The second, lidocaine, numbed the walls of his veins. We use that because the third, propofol, which induces a deep coma, can burn going in. Though it won't wake the patient, they may twitch, and that can make witnesses uncomfortable. The fourth, rocuronium, stopped Ted's lungs and heart. In between drugs, Sandy flushed the lines with saline. It was all quiet and efficient, and Ted was gone in less than five minutes. Sandy let more minutes pass before pronouncing the time of death.

I kept my face and my feelings neutral. But as I slowly came back into myself, what I felt myself reacting to wasn't

Ted's death. It was the process: how perfunctory it felt, how routine, how clinical. How chilly. The home already dismantled, the indifferent attendees, the proficient delivery of death. It was not at all what I had imagined when I committed to MAiD. What if every provision felt this sterile? Had I devoted myself to something that would make me miserable?

Then I met Joe.

CHAPTER TWO

Joe

Looking back now on the stream of emails that surrounded Joe's case, I am struck by how often I remember a provision one way—as simple or solemn—but my notes tell a more complicated story. In that way, I'm like everyone who remembers the dead: certain feelings and recollections rise up, while others fall away.

Joe had been a leather purchaser for Bata, one of Canada's most famous shoe manufacturers. He was opinionated—if a shoe didn't look good on someone, he'd tell them—but he wasn't dogmatic. He had married and divorced twice but stayed friends with his exes. He travelled the world, played golf everywhere he could, and, though he was diabetic, did five hundred push-ups a day. (He was proud of that, proud of his strength in general.) His dream for his retirement was to open a beach-shack bar on a Caribbean island, but he gave that up to be the caregiver for his mother, Sophie.

He bought a cat for her, Rolly, to keep her company when he was away on business. But it quickly became clear that the cat owned Joe. Rolly could sense when Joe's blood sugar was too low and would fret noisily around him, nudging him incessantly until he clued in and checked his levels.

When Joe was sixty-six, he was diagnosed with ALS, known more commonly as Lou Gehrig's disease. He'd felt numbness in his extremities for a while, and he knew it was something worse than diabetes. His golfing buddies did an Ice Bucket Challenge for him. Joe thought that was stupid; he worried they'd all have heart attacks.

Two years later, Joe's mother died, which made him feel even more desolate. Then Rolly began turning on him, scratching him unexpectedly. Some of the scratches led to infections, dangerous for a diabetic, and Joe knew he had to put the cat down. That felt like the final straw. He buried Rolly in the deep of night at the foot of his mother's grave, then came home and tried to join them. He injected himself with what he thought was a lethal dose of insulin.

"I had known for some time he'd probably try to kill himself," his cousin Wendy said years later. "He had it planned. He thought, while he could still manage his hands, that he'd overdose on insulin. He was frightened about it, though. I said I wanted to be with him, but he didn't want that, because that was illegal and would risk me being charged as an accessory to his suicide."

That first time Joe tried to kill himself, he panicked. He left Wendy a devastating phone message: "I screwed up. I didn't give myself enough." A few nights later, he tried again. The personal support worker who came regularly to bathe him heard him moaning inside and got the super to force the door open.

Joe was admitted to Birchmount Hospital (commonly known as Scarborough Grace), a towering red-brick building set next to a park. That stood out on my first visit to the hospital—how much more green space there was compared to my usual haunts, Toronto's three biggest hospitals, which stand in the concrete corridors of downtown. Joe was assigned to Dr. Stephen Barsky, the chief of psychiatry. Despite his impressive title, the chief had the demeanour of a buddy in hard times. Short and compact, he has an open manner that immediately puts you at ease; you feel ready to talk to him, to tell all. He must have been a godsend for Joe.

Once Joe was stabilized physically, Dr. Barsky transferred him to a geriatric floor (by this point Joe was in a wheelchair, a result of his ALS). There a combative patient assaulted him, and he was moved back to the safer, albeit locked, psychiatric floor, where he took up permanent residence in a room opposite the nursing station. He had his own bathroom and could mostly manage the transfers to the toilet seat. But his need for nursing help fluctuated unpredictably, and he knew that his disease would only progress. In the meantime, the psychiatric floor became his home, and the staff, his family—that will be important in a minute. By the time I met him, he'd been there nine months.

In late July 2016, not long after I'd attended Ted's provision, Dr. Barsky called me: his patient Joe had been following the legislation assiduously and was determined to be among the first to receive MAiD. But it wasn't an easy request to fulfill. Not only had Scarborough Grace never done a MAiD provision, assisted death was against its stated mission. It was rooted in the Christian ethos of the Salvation Army. The board would not be on side.

That wasn't going to stop Joe. He was going to die his way. If someone didn't want to talk with him about his death, he'd insist, "You've got to. You can't hide from it. This is about me. I want you to understand how I feel. I do not want to live like this." He spoke often about the physicist Stephen Hawking; the thought of living as Hawking did horrified Joe. "No way," he'd say. "I can't afford gizmos to help me talk." When one nurse on his ward disagreed with him, he actually chased her down the hall in his wheelchair, calling out, "Turn around, you've got to talk to me."

"Joe spent his last eight months teaching us what it was like to die," his cousin Wendy said. "Not in a cruel way. Just 'I want you to know this, I want you to understand'— how his body was failing, and his emotions around that. He'd say, 'Don't grieve for me. Support me. Don't feel sorry for yourself.' And he'd say, 'I'll be bugging you after I die.'"

Luckily for Joe, Stephen Barsky was not only his psychiatrist: he was his champion, his saviour—and his landlord. Joe had to present his case to the hospital board. He wanted MAiD in his home, he told them, and the hospital was home. A lifelong salesman, Joe knew how to make a pitch. He spoke passionately about what he would contribute to the understanding of ALS by donating his brain and spinal cord to the focused ultrasound research group at nearby Sunnybrook Health Sciences Centre. In fact, he told them, he had already made the arrangements. The cost of transporting his body from Scarborough Grace to Sunnybrook immediately after his death was two hundred dollars. He had the cash.

The board approved his request.

Dr. Barsky asked me not only to provide Joe's first assessment but also to be the lead doctor in this first—and maybe only—provision his hospital would undertake. There was not a moment of hesitation in my reply, even if there was a lump in my throat. I jumped.

Dr. Barsky met me at the door of Joe's ward—a locked ward, remember—and ushered me into a small interview room off the nursing station. He assured me that Joe's mental state and brain function were in no way compromised, despite his near-fatal overdoses, insulin shock, and depression. Dr. Barsky was proud of how Joe had bent the board to his plea and how the hospital had rallied behind the request. If I, as an external assessor, affirmed Joe's request, the next step would be an interdepartmental logistics meeting. Everyone would have to figure out, down to the smallest detail, how this would work.

Dr. Barsky walked me to Joe's room. Joe was in his wheelchair, waiting, casually dressed in easy-to-pull-on streetwear. He was well groomed, on the thin side but nourished, clean shaven with a ready smile and dancing eyes.

"How did you come to this decision?" I asked. He gave me the long answer.

When Joe was a kid, he spent a lot of time on his grandmother's farm with his brother and his cousins (including Wendy), racing each other through the fields, dodging cow patties. Joe had juvenile diabetes, so that was a bit harder for him than the others. Wendy had always been his favourite cousin; Joe would hold her hand as they ran and pull her up if she fell. "It didn't matter if we came in last," Wendy said. "Joe was always looking after people."

As adults, Joe drifted apart from his brother but remained close to Wendy. They called each other black sheep, because they both married and divorced twice. They joked that they'd be each other's date at weddings. He was a decent uncle to her son and daughter. And, of course, she was the one he called when his suicide attempt failed.

When he moved into Scarborough Grace, he became a favourite of the staff, who went out of their way to ease his challenges. He also had a small circle of old high-school friends who would take him out for the occasional haircut or meal. (Joe especially loved poutine and chocolate sodas.) But even those small pleasures were disappearing. He would ask a friend to take him out for pancakes, take one bite, and put his fork down. "It's not at all how I remember," he'd say. Toward the end, when he could no longer swallow and had a feeding tube inserted, he would still ask friends to bring him a hamburger or an Egg McMuffin. He couldn't eat it; it would just sit there. But he could smell it.

Now, Joe told me, all he saw ahead was inevitable decline and increasing dependency, and that was unacceptable to him. He was not in great pain, but he could feel the loss of strength, the creep of ascending paralysis. He already couldn't bear to call on the nursing staff to assist him to the toilet, even though his room was across from their station for that very reason. He didn't believe in an afterlife, but a friend had once told him that heaven was a fun neighbourhood bar where everyone he knew would hang out. He loved that image. He wanted to meet his mother and uncles at that bar and have a drink with them. Dr. Barsky and I approved his request and aimed for a date in August.

As the days passed, I kept busy with details. I had to get temporary privileges from Scarborough Grace (as all guest doctors do). I had to figure out my MAiD math, which was new to all of us. At that time, patients who requested MAiD had to undergo a ten-day reflection period, but when did that come into effect? From the day of request or the day of approval?

I also had to work through a bigger issue. To qualify for MAiD in those early days, a patient had to have a "grievous and irremediable medical condition," which was defined in four parts. One, they had to have a serious and incurable illness, disease, or disability. Two, they had to be in an advanced state of irreversible decline in capability. Three, their condition had to cause them enduring physical or psychological suffering, which was intolerable to them and could not be relieved in ways they found acceptable. And four, they had to be facing a reasonably foreseeable natural death. Quickly, we doctors adopted a shorthand for that last phrase: RFND.

The RFND clause was one of the legislated safeguards put in place to ensure protection of vulnerable people, those whose path to death did not conform to a strict timeline. People like Joe. A patient had to have a disease or disability that would be fatal "in a time in the not-too-distant future," and we doctors were charged with interpreting what that meant—weeks? months? years?—on a case-by-case basis. (We had to defend every MAiD death to a coroner. More on that later.) For Joe, Dr. Barsky and I agreed upon the most generous interpretation of *reasonably*. His diseases and conditions were fatal enough.

It was a maddening question for us doctors to parse, though—what did *reasonably* even mean? And to whom? We spent our own weeks, months, and years discussing and debating the RFND clause, and eventually the courts modified it. In 2021, the Superior Court of Québec ruled it unconstitutional and struck it. That same year, the federal Parliament passed Bill C-7, which removed the clause from the MAiD eligibility criteria.

But back to Joe. In those early days, the Canadian Medical Protective Association (CMPA), the legal go-to for Canadian physicians dealing with tricky liability issues, offered to help MAiD providers decide if a request satisfied the RFND clause. But I hesitated to consult them, because in my experience, their advice was inconsistent. I'd call them with a question, and the answer I'd get would depend on the individual who called me back.

Dr. Barsky and I, as early practitioners of MAiD, didn't want to depend on an outside entity to tell us how to do it. We didn't want to passively wait for approval. First, who knew how long an answer would take? Second, and far more importantly, we wanted to set the track. We didn't want to follow someone else's rule book. We wanted to—we had to—write that book for ourselves.

That flash of certainty I'd felt when I was on that treadmill watching the news—that I was one of the right people to do this work—was in part because I knew in my bones that my job as a MAiD doctor was not to focus on the constraints and restrictions and hazards and why-nots, but instead to show the way to yes. We physicians (and nurses, who would soon join the ranks) were the ones who had to make these decisions, because we have the expertise and skill that comes from providing patient care on a daily basis. Our concern could not just be about doing the job legally. Our concern had to be about doing the right thing for our patients, as we tried to do for everyone in our practices.

By this point, a Canada-wide network of physicians was coming together to support one another in those conversations (more on that later), and some of our earliest discussions centred on how to deliver the drugs: orally via a pill, or intravenously via a series of injections. We agreed that intravenous delivery was by far the better option: it was quick, it was painless, it was reliable. And we controlled it. We'd all seen patients vomit up pills. And what if a pill put a patient to sleep but didn't cause their death? Would we wake them up to give them another pill? In consultation with anaesthetists, MAiD doctors worked out the four drugs we'd require, and the doses of each. All of us wanted—needed—to be sure that we could do the job without mistakes.

The day before Joe's provision in August, I attended an interdepartmental meeting at Scarborough Grace—about twenty doctors, nurses, and other staff, plus the hospital's

CEO—to talk through the details. It stretched over two hours. Many of the questions were related to staff issues. Who should be involved? How many nurses? What if someone—a nurse, cleaning staff, anyone—was a conscientious objector? Would they be excused, and how would they become known to the MAiD team? Another big concern was how to keep the news of Joe's plan from spreading among the other patients on the psychiatric floor. Would they see it as a betrayal of a beloved fellow? Would it generate distrust and fear?

At the end of the meeting, Dr. Barsky took me to see the designated room, which had been prepared discreetly, well away from the ward. A volunteer board member had sourced paint, furniture, floor lights, and pictures. It was comfortable, warm, un-hospital-like. Dr. Barsky was proud of the effort, and I was touched by how many people had stepped up to make this possible. Joe's was a rare community, way beyond any psychiatric ward of my experience.

That night, I reviewed my notes about the drugs and their administration. Then I reviewed them again. I even drew pictures for myself, detailing which sized syringe was used for which drug, in which order. This was my provision. It was on me to do it perfectly. I went to bed, trying not to think about what a colleague had advised me about one of the drugs, propofol. "It's thick, milky stuff," he said. "You really have to lean on the syringe to push it through." I forced myself to sleep.

I was scheduled to meet Joe at eleven a.m. I'm an inveter-ate public transit rider, but that morning I treated myself to a taxi. As we pulled up, I saw a huddle in the parkette that sloped down from the front of the hospital building, thirty people clustered in the already torrid August heat. Instantly, I sensed that it was a service of sorts for Joe and headed over to join them.

He'd planned it himself. Beaming, he sat amid nieces and husbands and kids, nurses, social workers, and lots of cous-ins, including Wendy. Some of them didn't agree with MAiD, but they came for Joe. He liked to smoke marijuana; the nurses helped him take a few last tokes. Many of the party-goers, including Joe's friend of sixty years, Terry, would not follow us into the hospital—they couldn't face it—but every-one outside toasted him with his favourite drink, amaretto.

I broke off first and headed inside. The anaesthetist was waiting for me in the foyer. "Is this your first?" he asked.

"Yes," I admitted. I was relieved (I'd have help!) and also dismayed. Was my anxiety that transparent?

"Here's what I'd like to do," he said. "I'll draw all the drugs up and just hand the syringes to you one after another."

At that moment, the hospital's CEO rounded the corner, IV tubing slung over his shoulder. "Glad I caught you here," he said. "This is our new tubing. You only have to twist the syringes on, no needles. Thought you'd like to see it before you start."

I felt a surge of relief so enormous, I began to babble to them about a nightmare I'd had the night before. The dream recalled something that had happened when I was medical student. As punishment for not being skilled enough, my supervisor had sent me to start intravenous lines for a number of preoperative patients. The patients and the nursing staff were impatient to get to the OR, and I was clumsy and even more inept under that pressure. I woke up clammy from both the dream and the memory. I was determined not to repeat either; I wanted to give Joe a smooth experience.

By the time I got to the bright new room, it was packed with Joe's family, friends, and a great many hospital staff. All five of Joe's groomsmen from one of his weddings were there—they were passing around a wedding picture—along with one of his ex-wives. Joe lay in his hospital bed, which had been pushed into a back corner to make room for everyone. The mood was lively, a living wake. To Joe's surprise, his frail ninety-year-old aunt, a staunch Catholic, was also there. He had been sure she wouldn't come; he was afraid her faith would force her to damn his soul for all eternity. Apparently, she'd found a way to forgive him.

All heads turned as I entered the room—something I'd learn to get used to. I went straight to Joe. "It must have been hot for you in that parkette," I said. "What a crowd!" He was smiling, grateful and abashed at the turnout. I asked the required questions, a modified shorter version of the nine-point Mount Sinai document. Yes, Joe said, he wanted to go ahead.

Steady now, I told myself. All these people are here to witness an experience they have never had or thought much about. You need to slow down, explain what will happen. You need to prepare them.

I took a moment to introduce the team—myself, the nurse, the anaesthetist, Dr. Barsky. I explained how the procedure would unfold. "There will be four different drugs. I will administer them intravenously. The first is midazolam; it will make Joe fall asleep." I didn't name the next three; I felt it wouldn't register. But I told them what each drug would do. "His death will be peaceful and quick," I said.

The hospital chaplain, Pam Bauer, took over for a moment. In her mid-fifties, she was a bright light in the room, an effortless leader, clearly accustomed to guiding people through difficulties. She explained that she and Joe had picked out an appropriate song. She punched a button on her hand-held tape player. Monty Python's "Always Look on the Bright Side of Life" filled the room. Laughter— sort of. Then Joe said, "I am at peace." Reassuring words for all of us.

Pam asked if anyone had anything to add. Joe called out, "Let's get on with it!" Unprompted, Wendy clambered over the end of the bed, so she could hold her cousin as I administered the drugs.

I gave Joe the midazolam, and his eyes closed. I paused. "I'm not asleep yet," Joe intoned. Laughter erupted once again, real peals this time. I'm glad that was the last sound he heard.

I remember the anaesthetist passing me the other syringes, one by one. I remember that my hands did not shake. I remember that it was fast.

After Joe's pulse stopped, I waited. I listened for a heartbeat—none. I checked his pupils—fixed and dilated. I said to the room, "It's finished." The hush broke as people began to stir. One of Joe's friends approached me. "Is he gone?" she asked. I realized that I hadn't been clear enough. From then on, I learned to say, "Time of death . . ." and then name the hour and the minute. So everyone would know.

I sought out Joe's aunt to tell her that her presence had brought me joy, and I was sure Joe felt the same. Family and friends stayed on, unsure of what to do, or maybe not ready to go their separate ways. There was no rush to leave, no necessity to. It felt in many ways like any wake in a funeral home, old acquaintances being renewed, memories shared, no pain here. People were still chatting as my team and I quietly withdrew.

Wendy followed me into the hall. "Are you all right?" she asked. Only then did I begin to cry. The notion that she could see what I could not—that Joe's death was touching me as much as anyone else in the room—took me by surprise. I'm a doctor; I've seen death. Wendy had just lost her cousin, the friend of her life. Yet here she was, concerned for me.

It's not hardship that makes me cry. It's kindness. I'm the rock. But someone reaching out can crack me. The burden doesn't make my knees buckle. My knees buckle when someone lifts it. Wendy reached out to hug me, and I hugged back.

As I left the hospital, I felt no conflict in my soul. Sometimes people ask me, "But what about your Hippocratic Oath? 'First do no harm'?" Believe me, a lot of what physicians do is harmful. We can cause harm and perpetuate suffering, in the name of keeping someone alive. More chemotherapy. More radiation. Always one thing more to try. We're trained not to hear when someone says, "I want to go."

The difference with MAiD, of course, is that I am the agent of death. I am responsible for causing it. But that knowledge is the burden I agreed to carry. I don't think it's wrong, or immoral, or indecent. I think for the right people, it's the right thing to do. It's a kindness. But for me, it will remain a burden, always. To do this work, you have to be able to carry that with you, that you have actively caused someone's death. I carry it forever.

But that August day I was at peace. I rode the bus and then the subway back to my office. I watched the city flow by. I watched the business of life go on. I hadn't known Joe well, or long, but I had promised myself that his death would honour his life. I felt I had done him justice. Unlike Ted's death, which felt lonely to me, Joe's was the ideal scenario I'd imagined that day on the treadmill: a patient who was certain of his decision. A family who was supportive. An exceptionally responsive staff who knew Joe and cared for him as family. And a location that embraced the process. Everything about it eased not only his end but my entry into the practice. I thought all "my" provisions would be like this.

I was wrong.

CHAPTER THREE

Irene

If my belief that patients should receive MAiD from their family doctors was correct—and in those early days, I was stubbornly sure everyone soon would agree with me—then Irene was an ideal test case. She'd been my patient for fifteen years. I knew her story, her history, her family. (One of her sons was a patient of mine, too.) I had helped her through her husband's death, then watched her rise back up and rediscover herself. I saw her blossom with creativity, flirtatiousness, and adventure in old age. When she got cancer, I was there. And when she came to me to formally request MAiD, I'd already spent years listening to her lay out her wishes should she fall ill like her husband had, so promising her that I'd be the one to provide it was easy. She was the last person I expected to disappoint.

Most patients will never request MAiD. They want life, right to the final second, no matter what that end looks like. Only 2 to 4 percent of the general population will ask for assisted death. That's been statistically consistent across countries (including Belgium, Australia, and parts of the United States) and through the years it's been legal (since 1942 in Switzerland). The Netherlands, Canada's go-to resource, has held steady at around 4 percent for decades. Generally, people who request MAiD have thought it through from an intellectual and philosophical perspective. Many have lived through someone else's difficult or painful death, and they've suffered, too. They know what they don't want.

The most common reasons to consider requesting MAiD are the loss of the ability to engage in meaningful activities or of the ability to perform the activities of daily living, and the anticipation of pain and suffering. Pain management has gotten much more sophisticated in the last decades, and palliative care doctors are often able to assuage that fear. But the dread of being dependent on someone for care is not so simple to address with advancements in medical options. A patient can't stand the idea that they will need people, likely strangers, to feed them, dress them, and clean them up. They may also be afraid—depending on their illness—that they'll lose their memories and that they won't know their loved ones. That they'll become a shell of a soul in diapers with no quality of life. That they will no longer be themselves. And that is something that doctors cannot cure.

People want to preserve their dignity, to leave only good final memories for their family. That's certainly what Irene wanted.

We met in 2002, when she was seventy-six. I liked her immediately. She was vivacious, quick-witted, full of energy. Her eyes lit up with merriment as she chatted. She sparked with people from all walks of life. She drew you in, and you went willingly. She came from small-town Ontario stock; her great-grandparents had been early settlers. The family had had a store but lost it in the Depression. Irene joined the army to earn money for art college. That's where she met her husband, Arne.

Arne became a well-known artist and graphic designer. He was also a lifelong smoker. "He was never without a cigarette. Unfiltered," Irene told me. They had three sons, Jay, Steve, and Regan, and Irene put aside her own artistic ambitions to raise them. "A marriage with two artists would never work," she often said.

She loved life, and she channelled that love into her family. She bought cooking magazines and made experimental dinners on Saturdays. Friday was spaghetti night; they'd eat at the table outside in the garden and drink Arne's homemade wine. A feminist, Irene brought her sons to abortion-rights rallies. And leaving behind her artistic career didn't mean abandoning her creativity and passion for the arts. A fabulous boho-chic dresser (lots of head scarves and bangles), Irene designed her own clothes and sold some to a

Yorkville boutique. She borrowed armloads of books from a library in the Beaches neighbourhood and always took a book to bed. She loved Hollywood, the movies and the stars. She was the life of any party, the one who got things going.

When Irene and I met, Arne was already in treatment for lung cancer. But long before he got sick, he and Irene believed in the right to die with dignity. In 1985, their son Steve was the second person in Canada to be diagnosed with AIDS, and they'd suffered with him through his slow, painful death. That's when they joined an organization that was new in Canada then: Dying With Dignity. They remained strong supporters of it through the years and were advocates of living wills.

In the early stages of Arne's decline, Irene began making art again. I would see her in the cancer clinic at Women's College Hospital, sitting by his bed, sketchbook in hand. She had a facility for quick pencil sketches, which took three minutes or less. She caught her subjects in spontaneous acts: sitting on the subway, drinking coffee at a café, reading the paper on a bench. They were casual, informal, marvellously alive.

She began bringing her sketchbooks to her appointments with me, and we'd take a few minutes to leaf through them. I particularly remember one she'd done of Arne as he sat outside painting a winter landscape. Though simple, it was as vivid as a photograph.

But the sketches she made during the long days at Arne's bedside were quite different: stiller, sadder. Everything slowed down, her subject, her style. She'd zero in on inanimate things—the chairs, the equipment, the stretchers, the IV poles. In one precise close-up of Arne's hand, she drew his stretched skin, the IV line in his vein, the bandage covering it. These drawings radiated passivity, waiting, keeping watch. She was capturing Arne's decline through the details. Then I'd turn the page, and she'd be back out in the world: bus, subway, coffee, fluid again. Alive again.

After Arne died, Irene committed more fully to her art. She worked at it five hours a day. She expanded to watercolour, then oils. She travelled to Europe and the U.S. for courses. She joined the Toronto Watercolour Society. In her late eighties, she was entering juried shows and winning. She sold pieces, too. She loved her gang of artists, their parties, the wine that flowed.

In 2011, she underwent surgery to remove a cancerous tumour on her bladder, which was followed by six months of treatment. She sailed through. In 2013, she fell, breaking a wrist and fracturing her jaw. Soon after that she gave up driving; she took the bus or hitched a ride with friends to her outings and classes. But after a few more falls, she became fearful of being out on her own. Her independence was faltering.

In 2015, Jay moved into her house, to the upstairs flat. She was as clear with him and Regan as she was with me at our appointments: when the time was right, she wanted to choose the manner of her death. No lingering. She called the organization Dying With Dignity to learn what an advance directive was, and then Jay took her to her lawyer, where she signed one. While this could not authorize MAiD at that time, it gave Irene control over choices about life-sustaining treatment should she later lose the capacity to make those decisions. Her memories of Arne's death were etched into her notebooks: pus in his mouth, a stent down his throat to help him breathe. She did not want that end for herself. She wanted MAiD. And she was adamant, Regan told me later, that I provide it. "She didn't want a stranger to do it," he said.

At age eighty-nine, she developed a dry cough. She wondered if she was allergic to something in her painting materials. Then she had a coughing fit strong enough to shake loose her dentures. That got my attention. Irene had smoked for forty years but had quit in her mid-fifties. Was this a result of Arne's second-hand smoke? The long arm of her smoking history? I ordered a chest X-ray.

The radiologist told me Irene's right lung was collapsed. It could be pneumonia. It might also be a mass obstructing her airway. Two days later, the CT (computerized tomography) scan told us the story: it was a big tumour, the size of an orange. It was compressing the blood vessels around Irene's heart as well as her airway. It filled the space from her trachea to her spinal column. Multiple nodes were in the lung, suggesting the tumour had spread. More ominously, an enlarged lymph node below the diaphragm signaled metastases, meaning the cancer was spreading throughout her body.

Irene and her two sons met me to discuss options. Without treatment, she'd live three to six months. With treatment, she might have a year. After the usual gauntlet of oncologists, radiologists, and two biopsies, she knew she had the worst kind of tumour. Despite witnessing Arne's suffering, she opted for treatment: four courses of chemotherapy, given every three weeks. It was June 2016.

Her treatment did not go smoothly. Sores erupted in her mouth—perhaps from the chemo, or perhaps from her weight loss affecting her denture fitting. Her jaw ached. She stopped wearing her dentures. She lost her hair. She didn't want people to see her like this, so she hid at home. After a while, she missed her artist group enough to buy a wig and get back to work. They didn't care about her missing teeth. In August, as she turned ninety, she was finishing her last round of chemo. She was cheerful again, able to do complex crossword puzzles and paint three hours a day. She was working toward a show in November.

But as September advanced, so did her tumour, until her medical team deemed it "refractory to treatment." That's doctor-speak for, "The chemo didn't work. There's nothing else we can do." It's when we used to say, "Put your affairs in order."

Irene's mood plummeted. She fretted about being "off her game," a "pest." She needed help with bathing; that was embarrassing for her. Her appetite shrank. I prescribed Boost and an antidepressant. She kept reminding her sons, "If this gets really bad, call Jean. She knows what I want."

When Arne fell ill, they added a sunroom with its own bathroom to their first floor. Arne lived there until he was hospitalized. It was a lovely space, full of art and floor-to-ceiling bookshelves, overlooking their garden. Now it was her turn to move into it. She put aside her painting and her puzzles. Palliative care nurses began to visit weekly. Then, at the end of November, she fell four times in one week. Uh-oh.

We had a frank end-of-life conversation. She wanted to die at home. She signed a do-not-resuscitate order. But when I raised the question of when she might want me to assist her dying, Irene hesitated. That surprised me. She'd been so sure.

At the beginning of my long career, I did house calls. Then I stopped, far too busy with my office practice and the babies I was delivering at all hours. But for Irene, I did house calls again, twice a week. As January sleeted along, what I was seeing alarmed me. One morning she woke up thinking she was going to Ottawa to skate. With each visit, I could see her brilliance fading, her core self hollowing out. I knew this woman, her strong convictions, her attitude about life. But now she wasn't remembering things we discussed. She wasn't, Jay and I feared, remembering what she wanted.

As I said, I firmly believe a person's family doctor should be their final doctor. But with Irene, everything felt muddied: was my new role as her possible MAiD provider actually in conflict with my role as her doctor? There was a good chance that she'd soon coast to a natural death, without MAiD, so why was I so fixed on doing it before she lost capacity to consent? By urging her to remember that she wanted MAiD, was I honouring my promise to the woman I had known her to be? Or was I pushing a ninety-year-old woman to die, just to suit my mission?

I wrote up my consult notes, formally establishing Irene's eligibility for MAiD. I asked a colleague to provide a second assessment. I left Irene with a request form. She was set. But was I?

Uncertainty is not one of my default settings. I act first and ruminate later. Over time, though, my participation in MAiD would reverse that. More and more often before an assisted death, I would catch myself repeatedly combing through the details, mentally tussling with myself. That had consequences.

Like Irene, I came from tough stock. I grew up on a farm (hay, oats, wheat) outside of Cayuga in southern Ontario, fifty kilometres southwest of Hamilton. My parents, Wesley Bradt and Mary Bunn, had grown up on adjoining farms.

Dad was ten years older, so he first knew Mum as the kid next door; he knew her family story as well if not better than she did. In 1940, while living alone in Hamilton, she got in touch with him. She knew he was in the city working in the steel mill, and she wanted a connection to her farming roots. They were married within the year.

I now know how tough my dad's younger years had been. He was born in 1904, on a pioneer homestead in the then borderless Northwest Territories. After his mother died in 1906, his grandmother travelled west to bring him and his younger brother, Owen, back to the family farm, which adjoined the farm I grew up on.

Dad's father, also called Wesley (Dad was named for him), stayed on homesteading in western Canada, returning east only after his sons were grown. He became a hunter and trapper on lands of the Shawanaga First Nation, north of Parry Sound. The first and only time we visited him (and his second wife, Lucy, and their daughter, Adelaide), I was seven or eight. My memory of that visit is almost pure smell: pine trees, sunbaked granite, woodsmoke, warm cabin. Even today, I can still conjure the wet-dog scent of Rats, my grandfather's big terrier, and the dust of the endless car ride.

A few years after that trip, my dad brought his dad down to the farm to die. That funeral—the first one I attended—was held in the formal front parlour of the house, a room we rarely entered. I remember that it had its own separate door and its own organ in the corner. About the body, I remember almost nothing, other than he was laid out for all to see. I know that I felt no fear or sadness, only interest. Doctors need to hone a kind of detachment to deal with illness and death. It seems I had a head start on that.

I loved everything about our farmhouse, which stood atop a hill under a huge old oak. I felt a kind of magic in it. I loved that there was a large open dormitory on the second floor, with two staircases that led up to it. I loved that the grates in the floor up there let you peer down on the adults talking in the large kitchen. I loved the tin bathtub in that kitchen, which we used only once a week. (That suited me fine.)

My parents were a tight unit. They worked hard and never complained. Raised on the land and burnished by the Depression, they expected nothing other than what they could produce themselves. Dad was a man of few words, and on the surface anyway, Mom deferred to him. In particular, he didn't tolerate lip from children. He kept a black leather strap atop the refrigerator, but he never had to use it. When he eyed you over his glasses, the threat was enough to keep his three daughters in line: Mary Lou, the eldest by a year; me; and Joyce, three years younger.

When we weren't in school, my sisters and I worked hard in the fields, pulling weeds or riding on the combine to shuck wheat, oats, and clover, the dirtiest crop of all. We would load the wagon with bales of hay five rows high, climb on top, and ride like queens back to the barn. We were happy, busy children, singing in harmony as we sat on kegs of nails in Dad's truck.

At six, I staged my first rebellion: I refused to wear my hair in ringlets. My mother chased me around the table with a yardstick in hand and I finally stopped, overwhelmed by the futility of running nowhere. I'm a determined person, but once Mom put her mind to a task, I could never outmatch her steely resolve, or the swap of that yardstick. So, sigh, ringlets it was. In her late seventies, she became politically active, for a very pragmatic reason: she felt too many of her property tax dollars were slated for education in a county that was populated solely with retired old farmers. I was both amazed and proud.

Though deemed an excellent student, I still got into trouble now and again. My temper led to a lot of fighting, especially with playground bullies. I had an anger in me, begging for a righteous battle. At home, my father and I would argue about anything—whether only Churchill had been smart enough to see the war coming; if the Tudors were legitimate heirs to England's throne. Grudgingly, he and I found common ground, though it took me years to understand that provoking me was his idea of humour. No matter how heated the exchanges grew, my mother remained quiet. I suspect she was glad to see him so engaged with one of his girls, especially the one whose adolescent temper needed venting in ways other than through my fists. Afterward, she would calm me as I tearfully railed at how unreasonable and rigid he was being. When it came to my sisters' and my serious transgressions—staying out too late, skipping chores—Mum would know when and how to approach Dad, but never with us standing by.

I was the valedictorian in grade eight, already set on going to university (schooling stoked me). But I knew that was an extravagance beyond our means. The summer I turned fifteen, I took a job as an au pair at a cottage on Lake Joseph in Muskoka, the annual summer retreat of well-to-do Ontarians. In preparation, I sewed an entire holiday wardrobe.

Some holiday. I spent eight solid weeks working nearly around the clock—childcare, household cleaning, meal preparation—and earned a paltry $180. Never again, I vowed. Next I tried selling fruit out on the highway. (Dad would pick me up on his way home from carpentry jobs.) Then I tried picking worms at night on the local golf courses. To fill a pail with live ones, you had to be patient: hold, then tug. I was good at the tugging, not so good at the holding—few worms survived my frustration. In my last three years of high school, I landed steady summer work at a family-run lodge in Muskoka. I never spent a dime I earned from any of those jobs. Despite that,

I couldn't swing even the most affordable tuition, $450 for McMaster University in Hamilton. (I still marvel at the notion of student loans; borrowing money was out of the question for our family.)

Oh so tentatively, I raised the issue of tuition fees with my father. He was unmoved. "I have three daughters," he said. "Two are working and paying board. You are not. You can live here while you are in school, but I'm not giving you money. And I can't see what you think you are going to do. Your sisters have practical skills. You won't."

Admittedly, I'd once made the mistake of announcing to him that I wanted to be an archaeologist. His response said it all: "Dirt poor, digging in the dirt, a shovel over your shoulder." Few words, all of them choice. So I came up with a better plan: McMaster University had a nursing school, and the nursing school had a bursary that paid for all four years of enrollment. Finding tuition without incurring debt mattered more to me than whatever it was I would study. I applied for the bursary and got it. So a nurse is what I'd be.

Maybe it was fated. From the moment I started the course, I felt at home. The discipline, the workload, the physical demands—even the unspoken competition with the downtown Hamilton General Hospital's three-year nursing program—challenged me to succeed. There were only seventeen in our class, and we stood out in the hospital setting like sore thumbs. The nurse-trainees in the hospital's program scorned us as elitist. The engineering students on the university campus, who took organic chemistry with us, viewed us as exotic birds. It was all strangely exhilarating.

By January 2017, Irene was spending most of her time lying flat in bed. When she wanted to sit up, it took Jay five minutes to ease her into place. She wasn't interested in food. She needed help to put in her dentures and struggled to converse. Her hearing and eyesight were failing; she couldn't read, and she couldn't even listen to her Judy Garland and Liza Minnelli records.

She also was caught in a psychic loop. To her sons, she would say, "I want to go, I want to be with Arne." They'd call me. I'd ask her if she wanted to set a date for MAiD. She'd change the subject. I didn't want to push her; it was not my place to say, "Time to sort out your death!" I wanted her to give me the nod, and it worried me that she wasn't. The clock was ticking on her capacity to consent, and this faded person I was looking at was in danger of losing all connection with the vibrant person I'd known. But which one was now my patient?

I made home visits throughout January and into early February. On the last of these, Irene lay in her sunroom bed and talked about the final drawing she had made, a watercolour of her granddaughter (one of Jay's two daughters). Jay scrounged for it, then hung it on the bathroom door at the foot of Irene's bed. "That's what I want to look at as I die," she said.

I sat up. At this point I was doing MAiD two days a week, Mondays and Thursdays. Watching Irene gazing at her drawing, it felt like my last chance to engage the person I had known. So after she said the word *die*, I blurted, "And when will that be? How about Thursday February 17th?" To my relief, she agreed.

I sprang into arrangements mode. I ordered the necessary equipment to be delivered to her home. I booked a nurse to start the IV lines. I had the drugs sent to me. I made one last house call on the 15th. "Oh, I'm supposed to be dead," Irene said when she saw me. Not reassuring. But she laughed when I told her I was just checking in with her; the 17th was two days away.

That morning, I felt tense and unsettled. I'd hoped Irene would choose MAiD with calm certainty, but somehow we were stumbling into it. Was it even necessary now? She was surrounded by caring family, not in pain, not struggling to breathe. Was I doing this provision for me, to reassure myself that I hadn't waited too long, left her so vulnerable that she'd lost her sure footing?

Jay met me at the door. He and Regan greeted me warmly. We walked over to where Irene lay in her bed, an elegant head scarf tied just so, wig and teeth in place. I took her hand and asked again if she wanted this assisted death. "Yes," she replied. No confusion. No hesitation. I exhaled with relief and moved into the kitchen to prepare the drugs.

With everything ready, I stopped in the doorway and took in the scene. One of the great benefits of MAiD is that it provides time for closure. You can call a whole family into the room, to look at each other, to do this together. Is that what I wanted for Irene? Did I believe it was okay if her time on Earth was a little briefer so she could have this?

Irene was regal, alert, the centre of attention. Her soul was there; it had risen up to captivate everyone one last time. Jay, Regan, and Regan's wife took turns leaning close to her, murmuring private goodbyes into her ear. After she signed her consent form, her family toasted her with sake. I started the drugs, and softly she slipped away.

After Irene's funeral, Jay and Regan asked me if I wanted any of her art. I requested a sketchbook. "Which one?" they replied, laughing. "She has hundreds." A few weeks later, they brought two shopping bags full to my office and spilled them out across my desk. I chose two of the busy ones, the ones where Irene caught life on the run. Every time I leaf through it, I can feel her spirit in the rapid, fluid lines. Irene saw the beauty in life's fleeting moments, and she knew how to catch it.

As time passed, I expected my unease to dissipate. But it lingered. I had come to love that feisty, foxy woman. She deserved a death that fit her joyous life. But did I let my eagerness to give her that get the better of me? I thought Irene's would be an ideal example of my vision for assisted death, yet it felt far from perfect. Would it ever? Doing this work was going to be hard; I had no illusions about that. But if I felt this much doubt every time, it might be impossible.

As I mentioned, Canadian doctors never "kill" patients. We "provide" MAiD. *Provide* is a generous word. It suggests that you're giving someone a gift, doing them a service. That's what helps you sleep at night.

Sometimes you don't sleep, though. Then you have to get up, shove your doubt aside, and walk on. But it walks with you. It's behind you; it's over your shoulder. It's quiet. But it's there.

CHAPTER FOUR

Ashley

Ashley had a terrible, progressive disease, a rare genetic neuromuscular disorder that was never fully diagnosed or named. She'd lived with it since age one, when her walking was already notably unsteady. Her mother, Donna, knew something wasn't right and worried endlessly. The experts were certain Ashley would die because of it eventually, but no one could say how soon. What frightened her more was the stage before death: a vegetative blankness, which could stretch on for years. Bed-bound, without speech, recognition, or response. Total dependency on care round the clock. She was determined to avoid that. She wanted MAiD.

Her eligibility had been denied once already. The two thoughtful, thorough physicians who'd assessed her said she was only twenty-eight; years of life lay ahead for her. They couldn't see her natural death being "reasonably foreseeable" enough to satisfy the law's RFND clause. After all, no one really knew what her condition was. Maybe someone would find something to help her?

Doctors tend to be conservative in the best of circumstances, and these were early days for MAiD. Everyone was cautious. As well, Ashley lived in Collingwood, a small town about 150 kilometres north of Toronto, where everyone knew each other and their business. No one wanted to be held accountable for a "wrong" decision.

No one wanted MAiD requests to morph into doctor-shopping, either—going to physician after physician until you found two who gave consent. But Julie Campbell, a nurse practitioner who was then a MAiD intake coordinator for the provincial Ministry of Health and Long-Term Care, called me on Ashley's behalf. She knew that I was open to a wider application of the eligibility criteria than some. (There were so few of us doing this work back then; many of us knew one another.) She hoped that I could see "reasonably foreseeable" where Ashley's local doctors could not.

It's not that I said yes to everyone; I certainly did not. But I considered every case thoroughly, from every angle. If I decided that it wasn't time yet, which I often did, I would carry that patient's file open for months, even years. I would check in periodically to monitor any changes that would put them firmly on the road for MAiD. I wanted to support patients in their quest, not obstruct them. "Once I have you," I would tell them, "I have you until the end."

In June 2017, I took part in the first-ever national conference of MAiD providers and assessors. Part of that conference was devoted to drafting practice guidelines that would
make RFND clearer for both doctors and patients. We needed
a flexible definition of "reasonably foreseeable death" that
could stretch beyond a single year to two or five or even ten. It
was daring, yes. But it was necessary. The motivations that
drove patients who weren't actively dying to request MAiD
weren't always clear-cut or predictable.

Take cognitive decline. Doctors can't know how rapidly
it will progress. More importantly, each patient will react
differently to their decline. Losses that might not bother
one person might haunt and terrify another. One patient
might not mind being dependent on others; another might
loathe the idea. Which is more intolerable to you: being
aware that you are sliding into being incapable of doing
the things you love, the things that define you—or *not* being
aware? MAiD providers aren't there to judge; we are there
to listen. We need to assess each patient based on their personal definitions of "grievous and irremediable suffering,"
not just the words of the law.

Ashley was born two weeks premature, designated male and
given a different name at birth. The doctor who aspirated
fluid out of her lungs accidentally ruptured one of them.

Not a major complication, but it necessitated a longer stay in hospital.

From the beginning, Ashley missed critical developmental marks: walking, balance. Her mother, Donna, knew something was amiss. Eventually she took her to Toronto's Hospital for Sick Children (known as SickKids). Doctors there tested her for every known disease and genetic syndrome. The case was so mysterious that the genetic specialist, Dr. Ingrid Stein, presented Ashley's case at conferences all over the world.

The tests were painful, invasive, and sometimes terrifying. For one, Donna remembers lying on top of Ashley to keep her still while her (now ex) husband, Peter, held her head, so a needle could be inserted through her eye. But Ashley was a tenacious kid. She went to school with a walker and leg braces. She made friends; she did household chores. Writing was difficult for her; she never properly mastered it. By grade four, she was exhausting herself trying to walk, so Donna got her a manual wheelchair, which she lived in from then on.

Peter taught Ashley to shoot and took her to ride go-carts. She played sledge hockey in a local version of the Paralympics. She sold tickets at the Galaxy Cinema; she worked at Pizza Hut (where she once got locked in a walk-in freezer). She learned to drive the riding lawn mower. One afternoon as she was mowing, Donna was inside doing dishes. She heard the mower stop and looked up—no Ashley. Then Donna saw her dragging herself across the grass. Ashley had run out of gas, and no one heard her yelling. So she crawled.

When she was nine, the Make-A-Wish Foundation gave Ashley a six-thousand-dollar hand-propelled bicycle, which she used until she was eighteen. The foundation helped her have a lot of other adventures, too: she rode in a helicopter and a blimp; she visited a pit during the Molson Indy; she met the prime minister. She learned to drive a car and kept it up for about a year, until her eyesight began to fail. She was a loyal friend and a fierce enemy. When she loved you, she loved you through and through; but if you hurt someone she loved, she'd cut you off.

When Ashley was fourteen, Donna and Peter divorced. Their marriage had been "tumultuous," Donna said. "He liked everything perfect, and Ashley wasn't that."

At age fifteen, Ashley started experimenting with an emo look—she dyed her hair different colours, painted her fingernails black, wore eyeliner. She liked to wear girls' pants, instead of boys'; they were tighter and fit better, she told Donna. Then she started wearing a lot of pink. She never said the word *transgender*, and Donna didn't think it.

Ashley graduated from high school and went to Georgian College in Barrie, where she lived in a wheelchair-accessible room. One night she called Donna with an odd question:

could she break up with her girlfriend over the phone? Shortly after that, she sent Donna a text: she was suffering from body dysmorphia. She had always felt that she was a girl. But her disability had been so consuming, she'd been afraid to mention it. Admitting this now, and doing something about it, became crucial. It was one of the few things in her life she had control over.

Donna was surprised, but she took it in stride. She'd always had her son's back, and now she'd have her daughter's. Changing genders with the government requires a lot of paperwork—licences, birth certificates, health cards, etc.—and Donna dived in. Peter, on the other hand, could not accept Ashley's transition. They stopped communicating.

Donna took Ashley to an endocrinologist to begin a medical transition. To Ashley's dismay, the doctor thought she wasn't ready. She persisted. Six months later, the doctor started her on testosterone blockers and on estrogen. Ashley began to grow breasts, which pleased her. But she lost her upper body strength and gained weight. Donna switched her manual wheelchair for a motorized one.

"That just about did her in," Donna remembered. "It reminded her she was getting worse." Ashley's eyes developed an involuntary rapid movement, which made it too hard for her to play the online video games she loved, or even to watch TV. Swallowing became difficult, too. Throughout, Donna kept taking Ashley to doctors. She never lost hope for a diagnosis, which might lead to a cure. When Ashley aged out of SickKids, they switched to McMaster.

Getting to class and absorbing information was a strain, so Ashley cut back her course load. Going to the toilet in a wheelchair was always difficult; as her spasticity increased, it became even more so. She had a few embarrassing accidents, including one fall in a public washroom. She soiled herself and lay there for two hours before someone found her.

Ashley was twenty when she first mentioned the word *suicide* to Donna. Donna made sure Ashley went to therapy. She drove her to meetings of an LGBTQ2S+ support group. Ashley didn't warm to them. For one thing, they weren't wheelchair accessible.

After she graduated from Georgian College, Ashley moved back home. She had friends, but Donna was her best friend. "We did everything together," Donna said. But Ashley was becoming more and more reclusive. She wasn't happy, Donna could see that. She was frustrated that everyone she knew was moving on with their lives, while hers was getting smaller. The last type of exercise she was able to do was swimming, holding her legs together like a fish. Then she lost that ability. When she cried, which she did more and more often, it was scary for both Ashley and Donna, because she couldn't cry and breathe at the same time.

Her body ached constantly; she suffered crushing migraines. Donna bought her cannabis, hired a massage therapist, lobbied her doctors for new medications. Nothing helped. By this point Ashley could only listen to TV, and she played the same three movies over and over: *Black Hawk Down*, *We Were Soldiers*, and *The 13th Warrior*. Able-bodied people performing feats of strength. She'd fall asleep listening to them. "Her room was beside mine," Donna said. "I could have acted in them—I knew all the lines."

One of Ashley's main concerns was that her older brother, Jonathan, and her two half sisters from Peter's first marriage, Toby and Danielle, might develop her disease. She wanted to stay alive long enough for doctors to name what she had, so that if her siblings developed it, she could be their guinea pig. But after a doctor reassured her, "Your disease begins and ends with you," something changed in her. She stopped wanting to live and began wanting to die.

Ashley was determined to die as herself, though—in a woman's body. Donna took her to Montreal, which was then the only place in Canada performing surgical transitions. Doctors told Ashley the surgery was possible, but Donna was alarmed. The aftercare, to maintain the vaginal opening, took hours a day. It would be a massive undertaking for someone who was able-bodied; for Ashley, with her limited movement, it would be nearly impossible. Her despondency increased. "Every time she wanted something, she would hear, 'You can't,'" Donna said.

There was something else, too. In 2010, not long before Ashley began her transition, Donna had remarried, to a man named Paul. He was estranged from his own children, and at first he was supportive of Donna's. But as Ashley's dependence on Donna grew, so did Paul's resentment. "He was jealous of the attention I gave her," Donna said.

Paul didn't like it when Donna would get up in the middle of the night to clean Ashley after she had an accident. He didn't like when they had to race home from parties to help her. He wanted everyone to spend every weekend at his family's cottage, and he didn't seem to care that it wasn't wheelchair accessible. Eventually he built a ramp to the deck, but Ashley could never manage the shower. She had to wash outside with the garden hose. That was demeaning for her, especially so if she'd had a toilet accident. As well, Paul was uncomfortable with her transition; like Ashley's father, Peter, he didn't understand it.

When no one else was home, Paul began deriding Ashley. He'd mock her weight, criticize what she ate, be verbally abusive. He'd even trap her in her bedroom. Donna only found this out after Ashley was dead, from Ashley's personal support workers. While Ashley was alive, she'd made them promise not to say anything. She felt she was already too much of a burden for Donna; she didn't want to make things worse. She was a legal adult, so her PSWs had to comply.

Ashley began talking more openly about suicide. She could wheel her chair into traffic, she said; better still, she could roll it off the Collingwood pier and silently drown in Georgian Bay. At one point, she tried to slash her wrists with a knife, but she didn't have the dexterity in her hands to manage it.

One day Donna came home to find Ashley talking to a doctor. It was a MAiD assessment. Her daughter had applied for MAiD without telling her. "I went into a fugue state," Donna recalled. "I walked out of the house and just kept walking. I didn't know where I was."

Having a severely disabled child is hard on any family. Donna shouldered the burden literally: she lifted Ashley in and out of her chair so often, she needed surgery to repair both shoulders. When her kids were younger, Donna had enjoyed a busy career in radio advertising sales. But after Ashley came home from university, Donna gave up that job. Her daughter's disease had progressed too far; she needed help all the time. Donna began seeing Ashley's therapist, Alex, and taking the antianxiety medication lorazepam.

When the local doctors denied Ashley's request for MAiD, Donna was momentarily relieved. But Ashley insisted on writing them a letter, determined to change their minds. She needed MAiD now, before she lost her capacity to consent, before her disease took away the last vestiges of herself. She could no longer write on her own; she had to dictate her letter to Donna. This is some of what she said:

> I've been denied my choice to leave the world as I wanted to. I'm not sure if I conveyed why I want to die now. I've had enough of this life because it's not a life. I've had all the testing I want to endure. I live every day in pain. Some days I can't handle how much it hurts. I'm tired, I'm so very tired. . . . I'm scared I'll lose control. Even lying in bed gives me no relief from pain. I can't sleep more than four hours at a time. My brain is shrinking. I can't swallow without choking. I can no longer speak loudly. Soon I won't have a voice.

She had talked this through with her brother, Jonathan. Her life had narrowed to three options.

She could kill herself, but she didn't want her family to live with that stigma, and she was terrified she'd botch it.

She could do nothing and wait for her disease to engulf her. But that also would be horrible for her family, especially for Donna. Ashley's vegetative state would sap her mother's life, too. Donna would be with her round the clock, Ashley knew that. She wouldn't travel or spend time with her grandson.

As scared as Ashley was, she knew MAiD was her last best option—for her, because she could control it, as well as for everyone else. "I'm giving up my life so Mum can have a life," she had told Alex, their family therapist. "Please make sure she doesn't waste it."

Writing down her daughter's words, Donna heard the truth in them. Ashley wanted to go and, as hard as that would be, Donna had to help her. They looked up MAiD online, found Julie Campbell, and Julie found me.

We did her first assessment over FaceTime on our iPhones, a set-up that was then brand new to me. Ashley told me what the doctors had said: her heart and lungs were still functioning. They wouldn't approve MAiD until she was choking or could no longer breathe. "They don't want to be sued," she said.

I told her I would be willing to provide MAiD for her, and I would go to bat to establish the legitimacy of her request. But first I needed to confirm that her natural death was reasonably foreseeable, in its broadest definition. I needed backup from Ashley's long-time developmental neurologist, Dr. Tarnofsky, about the trajectory of her illness. He worked out of my old stomping ground, McMaster University Medical Centre in Hamilton.

Tarnofsky drew me a grim picture of Ashley's condition. She was, he said, "well past 75 percent" of her downslope to a vegetative state and total dependency. "Will that occur within the next five to ten years?" I asked. "Of course," he replied. Reassured that I could apply our broadest definition of RFND, I moved on.

Next, I called Andrea Frolic, the point person for MAiD provisions at McMaster. Did they have a facility that could provide for Ashley, who would be travelling about two hundred kilometres from her home? (Since Ashley had used that hospital for her care, it was considered her home base and could reasonably be called on to provide her with MAiD.) "We don't have one yet," Andrea replied, "but we're working on it." I recognized a kindred spirit—another person who didn't shy away from getting difficult things done. And I was proven right a few years later, when Andrea came back into my life for another reason. But for the moment, where could I provide for Ashley?

I steeled myself to approach the review team at my home hospital, Women's College in Toronto. I had worked hard to make my hospital a resource where community physicians could bring their patients. But Ashley was far outside their catchment, and like all hospitals, they were averse to becoming a "dumping ground" for those doctors or institutions who shied away from MAiD.

To my enormous relief, however, the team approved Ashley's request without protest and offered highly attuned, immediate emotional support for her family. We set a date,

January 16, 2018. Donna felt it was fate: Ashley had been born at Women's College. Now she would die there.

One of Ashley's regrets was that she never got to wear a prom dress. So for her last birthday, her twenty-eighth, her friends came to her party dressed for a prom. Ashley was in her wheelchair wearing a bridal gown she'd once modelled in a wheelchair-adaptive clothing show. She said she wanted to be buried in it.

When she wheeled herself into the MAiD room at Women's College on January 16, however, she was "full Goth," as Donna put it. Black dress, black leather boots. Her sister Toby had done her hair. Ashley wanted black lace over her face, so Donna had raced out to find a veil. She wanted to die in proper underwear, no Depends, so Donna had bought her sexy black panties, too.

As Donna, Jonathan, Toby, Danielle, and Donna's best friend, Jackie, filed in, I could see they were tense. They'd driven in through a snowstorm. They were worried about the timing. I assured them they could have all the time they needed. It turned out they'd had a terrible night: Ashley's stepfather, Paul, had railed at the whole family. Back in November, Donna had asked him to move out. She'd had enough, and she wanted to spend Ashley's last weeks focused on her. But he kept delaying. Ashley made it clear to him that she did not want him in the room with her as she died. But he'd driven down separately and was now outside the room, pacing the hall.

He wasn't the only one. Peter, Ashley's estranged father, had showed up, too. High drama, no serenity.

When Ashley was a child, one of the many physiotherapists had told Donna that it was great that Ashley was stubborn and tenacious; it would help her get through this world. And her stubbornness held to the end. A few times over the past six years, Peter had reached out to Ashley, but she wouldn't speak to him. When he heard that she was about to die, he'd redoubled his efforts. He wanted to apologize, to her and to Donna, and to say goodbye. He wanted to tell Ashley that he accepted her choice. He came to Donna's house, but Ashley wouldn't see him. Now he was in the hospital coffee shop.

Ashley didn't want to forgive her father. He'd made her feel guilty about her disability; he made her feel less than. And he'd hurt her mother. He wanted an eleventh-hour reprieve? Too bad.

Ashley's family lifted her onto the bed and wrapped around her shoulders a blanket decorated with pictures of Riley and Salem, her dog and cat. One of Ashley's sisters had *Black Hawk Down* cued up on her iPad, but for once Ashley didn't want to watch it. Her family was crying, and that made her cry, too. She asked for a lorazepam. Donna asked me if that was okay. "Everything she wants is okay, Donna," I replied.

Ashley was frightened. I could see that. But she was also determined. A few more family members had been mingling in the adjoining room; now they filed in to say their good-byes. Danielle's husband, Cameron. Jonathan's girlfriend, Megan. Toby's boyfriend, Mark. Mark said to Ashley, "I want you to know I'm going to take care of your sister. I'm going to marry her." Jonathan said, "I hope that's not your proposal." Ashley laughed at that.

Then it was time. My assistant—a smart, straightforward, no-nonsense nurse named Maria—entered, introduced her-self, and set about inserting the two required IV lines. Maria is one of those people whose steady efficiency and evident confidence in her own skills has a calming effect on those around her. I could feel everyone's shoulders relax-ing. I prepared the drugs. Ashley signed the consent form. Someone put on Ashley's favourite song, the Scorpions' "Wind of Change."

Donna sat on the bed. Jackie held one of Ashley's hands, Jonathan the other. After the first injection, Ashley fell asleep. After the third, Jonathan said he could feel her pulse stop. I let the family know when she was gone.

Later, Donna told me it was the first time she'd seen Ashley's face free of pain. But in the moment, she did something that startled me. She broke down, utterly. This woman who'd been Ashley's staunchest supporter in life, and her strongest advocate in her right to die, started wailing. "In my heart, I thought at the last minute she'd say no," Donna told me later. "She was my life. When you said she was gone, I was just consumed with anger. I felt all my hopes for her leaving me. I was just yelling at her, 'I can't believe you did this.'"

After a MAiD procedure, the doctor is required to phone a coroner, who confirms that the death is legal. In the earliest days of MAiD, a mere three coroners served the entire province, so I'd often sit for a long time with the family, or alone with the body, waiting for a call back. I tried to use that time to thank my nurses, to reflect on the patient, and to suss out whether the family wanted me to stay and talk or ebb away and leave them alone. (It could be awkward.)

The day Ashley died, the wait was excruciating. The entire time, Donna could not calm down. She couldn't draw a proper breath. She wouldn't let anyone cover Ashley; she wanted to see her face, even as her lips turned blue.

On the two-hour car ride back to Collingwood, no one spoke. It didn't help that they still had Ashley's wheelchair. The hospital didn't want it. So the family had to load it back into the van, and someone had to sit in it (Jackie volunteered). When they finally got home, Donna walked straight to Ashley's room and crawled into her bed.

A few days later, the crowd at Ashley's funeral filled the room and spilled into the street. Alex, her therapist, delivered a eulogy. Ashley could be petulant and demanding, Alex said. But also courageous, responsible, helpful. She lived her whole life with a disease with no name, and for much of it, in a body that did not match the person she knew she was. She dared to name that truth, and then determined to fix it. She lived not with a fear of death but a near-constant awareness of it. That gave her compassion for the suffering of others, a way of listening that others found reassuring. For years she felt suicidal, marked by stigma and shame, isolated and in despair. But when she learned that she could receive help to die, her mood lifted. She found a dignity that had not been available to her when she was facing a lonely, frightening death.

That's the thing about MAiD. It's one reason I can go on providing it. MAiD takes away someone's life. But first it gives it back to them.

CHAPTER FIVE

Education Complete?

By late 2016, I was in phase three of my self-designed MAiD program. I was travelling to Markham, a suburb twenty kilometres north of Toronto, twice a week to a family practice and palliative care unit at Southlake Regional Health Centre.

It was a lively place, to say the least. The small cadre of eight doctors provides both in-patient and out-patient palliative care, plus home visits and consultations to all the other services in the hospital, including paediatrics. They are a young, busy bunch of practitioners. They live in the community; they have children. They count on nurses to do a lot of the work in the clinic, and because it's a regional hospital with a large service area, they count on nurses in the community as well.

Much like at the cancer clinics in downtown Toronto, the Southlake nurses do the assessments, then fill in the doctors on what needs to happen. About the only thing they can't do is write the orders themselves. If you, a doctor, listened to them well enough, your work was done before you poked your head in to say hello to a patient. It was a high-demand, high-flow, intense place. I'd dictate notes as I ran from room to room and then come home, exhausted. And I was only there two days a week. It boggled my mind to think of the pressure on these doctors and nurses—and they were doing home visits as well.

Only one of their team, Dr. Howard Chen, had signed up to provide MAiD, and one day he asked if I could do an assessment on my way into the hospital. I readily agreed. No, I didn't know the country roads, but I had GPS. I was sure I'd find it.

Well. I drove and drove and drove, more and more anxious as my fuel gauge ran into the red. I don't recall the assessment, but I do remember that by the time I arrived, my tank was near empty. When I left, I asked directions to the nearest gas station. I made it—just. The metaphor nagged at me right away: my own fuel tank was empty. I was running on fumes.

And then my body made me face it. I herniated a disc. I didn't even do anything extreme—I simply stood up, and pain shot down the back of my leg. I knew immediately it was an L4-L5 sciatica. I couldn't stand on that leg. For one day, I stubbornly tried to keep up with the team, limping and leaning heavily on a walking stick. But getting into the car was a herculean effort, and I had to admit defeat. I put myself on temporary hold, gritting my teeth in frustration as my year of learning stretched into two.

Demand for MAiD was on the rise. It now occupied two full days in my week, and my slipped disc had cut short my time at Southlake. I needed to find my next "campus." In February 2017, I did: McNally House Hospice, a free-standing residential hospice located near West Lincoln Memorial Hospital in Grimsby, a town on the southwest shore of Lake Ontario, in the Niagara region of the province. The hospice operates as an independent, not-for-profit, community-driven organization that is well partnered with West Lincoln Memorial Hospital, Hamilton Health Sciences, and regional branches of Ontario's Home and Community Care Support Services.

Local family physicians have historically provided palliative care for their patients in and out of hospital and their collaboration with the Niagara West Palliative Care Team, McNally House, and the hospital elevated the collaborative efforts to an expert level. When I spent time with the team, it met every Monday and Dr. Denise Marshall, a palliative care physician with the Niagara West Palliative Care Team and McNally House Hospice as well as a professor of Palliative Care in the Department of Family Medicine at McMaster University, kicked off every meeting with an inspirational saying. The first time I attended, she quoted T. H. White, author of *The Once and Future King*: "Learn why the world wags and what wags it. That is the only thing which the mind can never exhaust, never alienate, never be tortured by, never fear or distrust, and never dream of regretting. Learning is the thing for you. Look at what a lot of things there are to learn."

I glanced discreetly around the room. Everyone else seemed into it. I, on the other hand, practically had to hold my eyeballs down to keep them from rolling. Surely this group didn't need inspirational prompts to validate their work.

As it turned out, the person who got inspired was me. I spent only a few half-days with Dr. Marshall and other members of the team—which includes not only physicians and nurses, but Home and Community Care case managers, bereavement counsellors, and more—over a two-month period, but I learned so much that I didn't even know I needed to learn.

The hospice served a population of about 100,000 in Grimsby and nearby community and rural areas. My gold standard would be six hospice beds per 100,000 people, but many big centres fall far short of that number. Toronto, by comparison, had 120 beds at that time for three million people, a much smaller ratio of beds per capita. Interestingly, and though some disagreed with me, my growing sense was that the availability of assisted dying was helping to increase palliative and hospice care services.

Those Monday meetings began at one o'clock, and the volunteers prepared a hot lunch to accompany them. At my first meeting, in addition to rolling my eyes, I declined the soup. Big mistake. Although I know well how sharing food can nourish the soul, this "family meal" reminded me how much can be accomplished in an easy atmosphere of chatting, of equal sharing, and of mutual respect. Everyone introduced themselves, as there were often newbies like myself in attendance, but each participant had space and time to discuss their patients and strategize solutions.

The independence of the team members was a marvel. They initiated the transfer of patients from homes to hospitals to hospices, without the usual administrative hassles we have become so used to. In addition, since the nurses and case workers shared their weekly records and care plans for all the patients on their list, it made anticipating and planning for what might be needed next much easier.

Statistics show that a dying patient usually spends fewer than three months in hospice. In my experience, it was more like ten days. But McNally House had one teenaged patient who'd been in the hospice for a year—not because he was dying, but because he couldn't move home with his mother until her house could be reconfigured to provide access for his wheelchair. The team was sure that was going to happen soon. In the meantime, if the hospice had to be his long-term care placement—well, they made it work.

The average length of stay at McNally house was seventeen days. To determine the right time to offer bringing a patient from their own home into the residential palliative facility, the team used a combination of lab results, clinical assessments, resources in the home, and often a decline in the PPS, the patient's palliative performance scale. The PPS, a diagnostic tool developed in the 1990s and now widely used around the world for both patients with cancer and other life limiting diseases, is comprised of five categories: evidence and activity level of disease, ambulatory ability, self-care, intake of food and fluid, and level of consciousness. Each category is scored out of 100 to give a rating that helps predict how long a patient will survive.

A PPS of 90 to 100 percent means that a patient is able to do everything on their own in spite of their illness (most often a cancer). At a PPS of 30, on the other hand, a patient needs help managing all self-care, is weak, bed-bound, and may be drowsy and lethargic. When that PPS is reached, we have learned over time that the likelihood of dying is usually within thirty days.

As so often happens in my experience, sharp declines and sudden changes often happen at night or on the weekends. A patient's pain may suddenly skyrocket, or they have bowel trouble, or they seem confused. How does the family caregiver manage? The team helps family members to anticipate those declines, they explain what to watch for; caregivers are prepared and know where and how to get help so no one is caught off guard, feeling helpless and alone.

When it is time for end-of-life care, patients can be moved smoothly from their home or hospital bed into the hospice, allowing both them and their families to have precious calm time. The whole family is being cared for until the end. The forewarning worked for everyone but especially, it seemed to me, for a family who was caring for a bed-bound dad or an increasingly confused mom at home.

I was there to sit with the staff, review the orders, change some prescriptions, and attend to the patients. But mostly I listened and did a lot of nodding in agreement. When I visited patients in their rooms at McNally House, I felt comfort and peace. Their families felt at home; they came and went freely. People were here to die, but no one was unattended, no one was afraid. There was sadness, of course, but also space for a lightness of spirit, tranquility to chat about the daily minutiae of life, laugh a bit, detach from gloom and helplessness.

Another remarkable element of the team was the cadre of some 130 volunteers, who were organized as tightly as the staff. They covered four-hour shifts from eight a.m. to eight p.m., during which they did meet-and-greets and orientation for patients and families. They assisted personnel, managed visitors, and generally made life easier for both staff and patients. Denise said that she couldn't do what she did without their help. They also brought in an endless amount of baked goods—and that Monday meeting soup.

My favourite part of the time I spent at the Grimsby hospice was doing visits out in the country with Denise and her dedicated team nurse. No GPS for those two. They knew every farm, all the backroads, the whole county's history. They reminisced about things they'd had to do, back in the day, to get the old farmers—diehards—into hospital. They had bone-deep knowledge of the histories of their people, and nothing but admiration for their tenacity.

Of course, those Grimsby farms reminded me of the ones I'd known growing up. In 1961, as I was starting university, my father, then fifty-seven, had a heart attack while doing heavy labour, repairing machinery at a steel plant. He was brought to the hospital where I worked as a volunteer. He was filthy with the oil and grit of the job, and I'll never forget the compassion of the head nurse as she bent over him, calling the orderly to come and bathe him on the spot before he was seen by the doctors. His pain was abdominal, but it was his heart that was critical. It took two days to sort it out, and we were staggered to come into his hospital room and see him sitting up with an oxygen tent covering the bed.

He spent six very impatient weeks in bed, and when he was released, he was ordered to cut back on his workload. Mary Lou had moved to California by then, and Joyce had gotten married. (I made her entire trousseau myself, from a high-end *Vogue* pattern book. We were children of the '40s, remember.) So as Dad improved, he and I fell into lockstep, doing farm chores together on weekends and harvesting in the summer.

The barn housed pigs, fed continuously for six weeks to fatten them for market. One April day, we were in there popping the glass windows out of their frames to let in spring air. I inadvertently stepped into pig manure and sank up to my waist. I can still hear Dad laughing uproariously. Eventually, he demolished the old farmhouse and built a retirement bungalow for my mother and him, where he lived until he died. My mom stayed on living there—first alone, then with her second husband, and then alone again after he, too, died.

I was sailing through nursing school, or so I thought. But in my third year, when we were deep into providing actual nursing care, one of the instructors called me into her office. She told me to sit down and then she raised the question of my suitability for this profession. She catalogued my many errors. For one, my hair-braiding skills were abysmal, and my impatience with these small but essential tasks of patient care were blatant. As well, I had made a serious mistake with a drug dosage, for a patient who had come from the city jail. Perhaps I had been rattled that he was handcuffed to the gurney. But my mistake had reverberated through the rank and file of our rival hospital nursing students, and the reputation of the university nurses was tarnished.

"Wouldn't you be better," my supervisor asked me, "in another, less care-based occupation?"

My retort surprised even me: "Over my dead body will you get me out of this program!"

Underneath, however, I was panicked, and my panic led to a despair that was uncharacteristic for me. I'd invested three years; leaving the program screamed of failure in my mind. Besides, what else would I do? I didn't see any other options. The dark blue walls of my hospital dorm room, a gloomy single, were a concrete manifestation of my mood. Ever driven by action, I requested a room change, and somehow it worked. I felt that if I could control moving rooms, I could control everything, and my new yellow walls helped goose me back into business. It wasn't that easy, burying the misery, but in the end, I steeled myself to finish, no matter what the program demanded.

I graduated in 1965, into an Ontario that desperately needed nurses. (It still does. Even before the pandemic, Ontario had the fewest number of nurses per capita in the country.) My first job was as a charge nurse—a scheduling and overseeing job—in the same hospital where I'd been a not-always-appreciated student. That felt like a victory, even if the job description put me firmly into the ranks of an administrator and a desk nurse, not a "real" one from the hospital-trained corps.

When the opportunity arose to become the visiting nurse-liaison between the hospital and the Hamilton community, I jumped. I loved the independence. I loved covering all parts of the city. Quickly, I saw the real-life struggle of people out there on their own. I visited homes where the cleanest thing in them was the daily newspaper I carried with me, the only thing I dared put my bag down on. My farm-strengthened back came in handy when I had to do a bed-bath for someone whose mattress was on the floor. I learned to hate the smell of Dial soap, which had flooded Hamilton homes via some weird freebie offering. But I meshed with so many people and came to love them. Forty-five years later, I still have Mrs. Smith's recipe for spaghetti sauce.

My next move came via Dorothy Pringle, a friend and colleague who'd graduated a year ahead of me. She had taken a job at the Lakeshore Psychiatric Hospital, a sprawling collection of century-old red-brick buildings set in lush parkland on the waterfront. The hospital was launching an entirely new aftercare program. Dot was running things on the women's side and had put my name forward to run the men's. Not only would I care for patients after their discharge, I'd frame and manage the whole program, including coordinating with the staff and running group meetings. It would all be on me.

Psychiatry would be a leap. In nursing school, my only psychiatric training consisted of two months in a rambling facility on the Hamilton escarpment that, in some moments, led me to feel I was working in a genteel version of *The Snake Pit*, the turgid Olivia de Havilland film from 1948. Not a reassuring recollection, but I wanted to be in Toronto for a more selfish reason. My new boyfriend lived there. We'd met in my fourth year of university, while I was still on the high of being crowned McMaster's Snow Princess. (That's a story for another time. I will admit that I sewed, by hand, my black-velvet evening gown.) And the yacht club on Toronto's islands had wonderful eight-metre sailing craft, and I was determined to learn to crew those magnificent vessels.

I needed an apartment, which meant I needed furniture, so I scoured our basement. I found an old cupboard, which I stripped and then finished into a dresser. Dad helped me fashion a bed frame with a flip-up back that converted to a couch. I sewed cushions to sit on by day and sleep on by night. I sawed several inches off the legs of a table to make a coffee table. It was also my dining table—I sat on a cushion on the floor.

For my first and last month's rent—five hundred dollars I did not have—I went to the nursing director. (Dad had not changed his mind on the subject of loans.) "I need an advance on my salary," I said, a firmness in my voice not felt in my quaking knees. At first, she was flabbergasted. That was a lot of money. I stood my ground. She offered to run it past the chief of psychiatry, Dr. Ron Stokes, and to my amazement, he lent me the money. I paid it back, gratefully, with my first paycheque.

My learning curve was an arrow straight upward. I learned to co-run group therapy sessions. I learned never to sit with a paranoid patient without a clear exit path. But I always felt I was scrambling to catch up, and I was defensive about all the things I didn't know. I acted confident and thought I was getting away with it—until two years later, when Barbara, one of my group co-leaders, a wise, British-trained social worker, remarked that the chip on my shoulder had finally melted away.

In 1968, I was offered the job of head nurse at the Clarke Institute of Psychiatry (now the Centre for Addiction and Mental Health, or CAMH), for one of their small inpatient units of ten beds. The unit had nine nurses (including me), two social workers, three resident psychiatrists, two occupational therapists, two psychiatric resident doctors, a secretary, a ward clerk, and the unit chief. That sounds like a lot of psychiatric muscle, but we needed every ounce of it to provide the proposed outreach services to the Toronto borough of East York's youth and families.

My job was to organize the nurses' twelve-hour shifts in the hospital and still leave room for their work outside it—in small group settings with kids at risk, with immigrant groups, with new mothers or teachers. It was a thrilling idea: a team of nurses behaving in new ways, responsible for their own learning, and for identifying and exploring opportunities with no guideposts or regimens. Grassroots, ground-up, blank-slate stuff. We would see what needed to be done, and we would figure out how to do it.

I was supposed to be the overseer, the backbone of the team, the presumptive leader. But even as I was hiring the nurses, they seemed braver and smarter and more embracing of risk than I had ever been. They became proficient as therapists, group facilitators, marital counsellors, and outreach workers. They invented new programs and services. They applied their remarkable expertise to assist outside agencies, while I settled into a routine that was comfortable and rewarding.

But I had overlooked one critical detail: the program was conceived as a five-year trial. In order not to become self-perpetuating—*indispensable* was the word we used—it had built in its own termination via a sunset clause. Three years in, I realized I was about to lead a planning meeting about the next two years of programming—and about how the program was to end.

To end? I went cold. My perfect world had an end date? What would I do then? I sat in that meeting and heard nothing. But I knew in a flash that I had come too far and done too much to return to any regular—hospital-bound, subservient-to-doctors—practice of nursing. The obvious, the only, solution: I had to become a doctor.

McMaster, my alma mater, seemed an obvious choice. Back I went for an interview, but I was dissuaded. The medical school program, new at that time, was directed toward attracting candidates already accomplished and successful in fields outside medicine. A graduate from nursing school, even a McMaster alumna, didn't cut it.

I waged a full campaign to get into my next choice, the University of Toronto. I enlisted the professor of psychiatry and my chief of service, both men, to write letters on my behalf. Their efforts made a difference. U of T offered me a place—but only if I could pass the prerequisite organic chemistry and mathematics requirements, two subjects I'd strenuously avoided throughout my education. That summer I did both courses at the University of Western Ontario (now Western University), in London, in a mad, six-week rush. I've never worked harder in my life, but I achieved the required grades by the skin of my teeth. In September, I entered U of T. Three years of med school and one year of internship later, I became a family doctor, and I stayed one for forty-five years.

My nurse's training never left me, though. Even though I don't think of myself as particularly compassionate, my memory of that ER charge nurse gently laying her hand on my father's grimy shoulder as she called for the orderly to come bathe him gave me my model for good care. So I am proactive. If a patient's bed needs stripping and the nurses are too busy, I'll do it. I get my hands dirty. I sometimes see that as a character flaw, because it's gotten me into trouble. But impatience, I've learned, can also be a virtue.

On those farmhouse visits, I saw a lot of makeshift care for elderly, addled, and/or bed-bound parents. But that duo were unfailingly considerate and always thought to ask their patients' caregivers (as always, usually daughters) what was hard for them. These were people who didn't share their troubles easily, but they shared them now. I was reminded again and again of my early days as a visiting nurse. But I had never felt so wrapped in the power of good as I did when I was with these two women. It was a rare privilege to be an observer to their skill, to see what can be accomplished when end-of-life care is approached with this depth of respect.

Tellingly, we never discussed MAiD for any of these patients. The Niagara West Palliative Care Team's formula was working: it helped people die on their own terms, without any added intervention. If all doctors and nurses had such a team and resources at their fingertips, I pondered, would we need MAiD at all?

If only. In truth, only a small proportion of Canadians will ever opt for an assisted death. The vast majority of us will want and expect the kind of end-of-life care that was so beautifully observed in practice in that unit.

It was the perfect place for me to end my year of independent learning. Excellent palliative care is the ideal, and I saw it in action. But seeing the ideal also let me see the gaps more clearly—or rather, the gaping divide between ideal care and what far too many people were getting. There are so many reasons for that divide: too many people in the cities, too few in rural areas, not enough money, too many people living alone without help or connection. And far too much neglect of the elderly, from both our governments and our youth-obsessed, time-strapped society.

The warehousing of our elders—it is the last and most-feared option. Who hasn't heard, "Let me die before you put me in a home!" from a friend or relative? Yet for most of us, it's the best bad choice. Medicine has directed its resources toward cutting-edge acute care, and one cost of that (unless your family is sitting on chests of gold) is shabby, under-serviced and under-resourced long-term care facilities. The COVID-19 pandemic brought that shame to the forefront in 2020, as elders died in disproportionate numbers. Canada's population is aging. Unless things change, exemplary chronic care, not to mention model palliative care such as that I witnessed in Niagara, will be out of reach for many, perhaps most.

My time with the Niagara West Palliative Care Team showed me what my challenge was and my goal.

I was evolving the template of how I would approach MAiD assessments.

The standardized form for a palliative care consultation would serve as my base, as it had done during my time in the active treatment clinics. That template includes a complete history of the illness and treatments, a thorough physical assessment, and review of past medical issues. It has a rating system for symptoms such as breathing, elimination, pain, mood, appetite, and fatigue. It assesses a patient's social history and current personal and spiritual supports. It plumbs the patient's and family's strengths. And since all my work is outside of hospital, I need to assess those community supports as well—nursing, personal care, disability aids beyond family care. Have they been utilized? Do they exist? I consult with their doctors, who have known them over time.

And along with that knowledge comes the exploration of the patient's request. How do their values, fears, and expectations frame the request to have help to die, on their own terms, in their own time? How does the sense of life's purpose, the exercise of control of their end, or the need for dignity lend credence to their ask? Who supports them? Who obstructs?

The creation of a plan of action is a dialogue between the patient and me that leaves the patient in control. Often that fact alone is enough to lighten the load of fear for them and it grants them not only peace of mind but sometimes lets them continue that fearful journey longer, knowing they can say, "Now is the time."

I would never rush anyone into MAiD—I would discover why they were asking for assistance to die, and why now. I would ferret out other possible options, and if the patient refused them, I would seek to understand their objection. I would see them, and hear them, and when the reality of decline and suffering dictated the choice, clearly in their hands, I would step in to end their lives.

CHAPTER SIX

Sheila

In January 2017, six months into my own MAiD practice, I hit my first serious roadblock. Not only has it had a lasting impact on me, but the issues raised are vital ones for legislators who determine how we handle MAiD requests from patients who have early stages of cognitive loss. Our aging Canadian public wants to preserve their dignity and control their destiny, even, indeed especially, if they are no longer sentient. We find ourselves in continuous pursuit of legal modifications.

Sheila was only sixty-eight, but she'd been diagnosed with primary progressive aphasia, an aggressive form of dementia. She was already losing words. Her mother had had Alzheimer's, so Sheila knew what was coming, and she wanted MAiD while she was still able to consent. Her partner of six years, a retired dentist named Alan, supported her request. But her adult daughter, Lisa, emphatically did not. And Lisa had Sheila's medical power of attorney.

When we met in person, Sheila showed none of the more blatant signs of dementia: uncertain gait, reaching out for a steadying arm, indifference to personal appearance, fear of encounters. She was perfectly groomed, carefully and elegantly dressed. The personification of togetherness.

Lisa, on the other hand, was visibly upset. I learned much later that Sheila had not told Lisa about this appointment— and she'd made Alan promise not to tell, either. But Lisa had found out and felt she had to be present. Lisa and her brother, Brahm, didn't trust Alan. Alan could feel that mistrust. Alan thought Lisa wasn't doing enough to care for Sheila; Lisa and Brahm thought Alan was manipulating their mother, keeping her away from them. There were suspicions on both sides that money was a motivation. Though I didn't know all this then, I felt the tension.

It didn't rattle me too much. Children often disagree with a parent's choices and motives. Over the long course of my practice, I'd been in the middle of many of these disputes, and I prided myself on my negotiation skills. What perplexed me was that, for different reasons, neither Lisa nor Alan was confident that Sheila would be able to express her wishes adequately. Were they being overprotective? Was Sheila's togetherness a careful construct? I asked to interview her alone.

She became visibly nervous. She spoke haltingly, afraid that I wouldn't understand her or would impatiently hurry her along. I reassured her that I would give her all the time she needed. There was no rush. She had my full attention.

Sheila had a large, sophisticated vocabulary, which was a source of pride for her. But as far back as fifteen years ago, she began noticing that she was saying the word *thing* (instead of the word for the object itself) far too often. Now the loss was expanding. She was stopping midsentence and searching for the word she wanted. She didn't understand the use of common objects. Not only could she not remember the word *carrot*, for example, she needed prompting to remember that it was for eating. Her short-term memory was also failing. She was struggling to follow instructions in sequence. She was getting lost on roads she once knew well. And she was deeply embarrassed by it all.

Wait a minute—Sheila was still driving? "I only go to the same places," she explained. "If I get lost, I stay calm and drive around until I see a place I know. Or I call my son, Brahm. I tell him the street names where I am and he guides me home." Staggering, I thought, the strength of her desire to hang on to herself was so fierce. It gripped me with both sadness and admiration for her grit.

Throughout our interview, Sheila never let her gaze leave my face. I could see her constantly checking that I was not only registering her story but also acknowledging her misery. (I was; it was painfully obvious.) I concentrated on listening to her few words, giving her time to frame them, resisting the urge to jump in and do it for her. The background I could get later. I needed to *hear* her. "It is . . . going on . . ." she said, fighting through the pauses, "and I am . . . afraid."

Doctors are trained to listen for clues so we can frame a diagnosis and a treatment plan. If the treatment isn't exactly right at first, that's fine, we can always readjust the plan. Action is the goal, not reflection. It's easy to miss the nuances of a patient's story.

But helping someone to die, I was learning, required a different tack. To do it well, I needed to dive deep into a patient's motivations, to listen for their soul.

I think I saw something of myself in Sheila's determination to carve out her own destiny, no matter the obstacles. She was born in Montreal to immigrant parents. Money was a struggle; sometimes they went without heat. At age fourteen, she quit school to help support her family. For the rest of her life, she would talk about how she wished she'd been formally educated. She made up for it by becoming a fierce autodidact. She read books and newspapers voraciously; she raced through crossword puzzles. At nineteen, she married her boyfriend of three years. They moved to North York, outside of Toronto, where he started a painting and contracting company. Sheila, who prided herself on being a quick study, was the office manager part-time. Confident and beautiful, she moved easily into becoming a vivacious hostess who loved to entertain her wide circle of friends.

"She threw the best parties," Lisa later told me, "and she threw us the best birthday parties." Sheila also loved going out: to movies, plays, the symphony. She was determined that Lisa and Brahm go to university. "There was no *if*—it was *when* we went," Lisa says.

In 1998, Sheila's husband got stomach cancer. The family tried everything: specialists in Toronto, a trip to Sloan Kettering in New York, even an experimental program in Japan. But the cancer was unstoppable—seven weeks after his diagnosis, he was dead. "My mother fell apart," Lisa says. "She went from being a bold, extremely independent, 'I can do anything' person, who would go to bat for anyone, to totally incapacitated. She couldn't decide the simplest things, like where to meet a friend for lunch."

Sheila moved in with Lisa and Lisa's new husband and stayed seven months. Even after she bought a condo, she'd be at Lisa's every afternoon. "I go back now and wonder, Were those already signs?" Lisa says. ("It was a long time to live again" was how Sheila put it to me when we met.) Lisa and Brahm both had children; Sheila doted on them. Eventually, she dated, she moved in with a man, they broke up. Then in 2011, she met and soon moved in with Alan.

"The first two years," when she felt they were equals, "were very good," Sheila told me. "The last four years, not so," because she felt she was a "burden," who "had no purpose." She'd experienced the past two years as a nightmare, a ceaseless struggle to find words. Alan was a runner, a skier, a traveller. Sheila didn't want to do those things anymore. She tired easily. She was tuning out.

She and Alan had discussed MAiD—a lot. "Neither of us wanted to stick around if we didn't recognize anyone, couldn't talk, couldn't participate in life," Alan told me. "We'd both had mothers with dementia."

Sheila had taken her first Montreal Cognitive Assessment (MoCA) test back in 2000. It's a simple, fifteen-minute, pencil-and-paper quiz, which allows quantification of memory and reasoning, to assess mental capacity. (It's the test Donald Trump crowed about passing, as if it were the LSAT, the MCAT, and the GMAT rolled into one, when in fact one question asks you to identify a picture of a tiger or an elephant.) In 2000, her results were normal. From 2012 to 2014, her results showed mild cognitive decline.

But she'd not submitted to a new MoCA in three years, nor to SPECT—single photo emission tomography, a test that enables doctors to see the specific areas of the brain that are malfunctioning. Most doctors would want to administer one at every follow-up. Tracking changes in a patient's brain is incredibly helpful in predicting the progress of disease or assessing medications to stall it. But Sheila had been too ashamed—or too scared—to confirm her decline, an avoidance that's all too common among dementia sufferers.

Despite her struggle to speak, I heard the terror in Sheila's request for MAiD. She did not want to end up wordless, unable to express her desire to "be gone." If she wasn't so afraid that she'd "botch it," she told me, she'd take her own life. At that point I'd only been providing MAiD for six months, but already I'd heard this suicide option a lot, from patients who feared it was the only escape from the pitiless suffering they were enduring over time. It surprised me, however, that this delicate woman was considering it. Again, her palpable determination gripped me.

Was this because I, like many of us, fear dementia, a future without my mind, of being me but not-me? Probably. I'm over eighty. I ran the Boston Marathon nine times before COVID hit and won my age class eight times. I bake huge trays of lasagna for frequent, chatty dinner parties I host. I throw an annual Christmas bash where my guests sing carols and recite poetry. I have a country place on Georgian Bay where I kayak, garden, and turn wood. If all that narrows and fades to grey, if I end up like a still-alive butterfly specimen, writhing silently on its pin, I don't want to stay here, either.

But as willing as I was to provide MAiD for Sheila, her request faced major hurdles. The first one was her daughter. To Lisa, who would control Sheila's medical care should her mother become incapacitated, Sheila was still managing well, still engaged, still present for her children and grandchildren.

The second hurdle was legal: that RFND clause again. We've adapted the rules since 2017, but back then, to qualify for MAiD, a patient's natural death had to be reasonably foreseeable. Sheila's wasn't. Unlike Alzheimer's, which attacks the whole brain and ends up shutting down the body, aphasia initially only affects parts of the brain. From the neck down, Sheila was in perfect health.

Which is why the third hurdle was moral. Sheila could live thirty more years—trapped in her well-functioning body without words. She didn't want that, so I didn't want that for her. This was a hard one. I couldn't do this alone. I needed Sheila's doctor on our side.

That was hurdle number four. Sheila's doctor, Sandra Black, is one of Canada's foremost researchers into Alzheimer's. Her contribution in this field is legendary. I often joke that her CV must list fifteen hundred publications. She'd been seeing Sheila at Sunnybrook's neurocognitive clinic every six months since 2015. To me, Sheila's disease was advanced, causing grievous suffering with a clear trajectory to death. But would a doctor who'd devoted her life to the treatment of this fearful affliction agree?

The issue was much bigger than just Sheila's case. How to handle cognitive decline was and continues to be one of the biggest debates in MAiD, even after all the changes of 2021. (More on those later.) But back in 2016, I needed a bargaining chip. I told Sheila that if she agreed to be retested, it would document her further decline and help justify her request. She agreed. Thus armed, I called Dr. Black.

She's a formidable, academically intimidating woman. The first time we spoke, I was midway to the hospice in Grimsby, one-hundred-odd kilometres west of Toronto. "I'm driving, but I'm fine to talk," I said breezily. "I'm on hands-free speakerphone."

"Pull over!" Dr. Black ordered. "Are you aware of the errors in judgment drivers make because they are inattentive to the conditions around them as they talk?"

I looked across the four-lane highway at the other cars whizzing by me at one-hundred-plus kilometres per hour. Suddenly, I was acutely aware of the hazards of being inattentive—to Dr. Black. I said goodbye, took the first exit, and called her back from the dead end of a country-road bypass.

I told her my impressions of Sheila. She was way ahead of me. For an hour, I sat by the side of that country road trying to keep up as Dr. Black gave me a crash course: which part of the temporal frontal lobes were involved with word association, memory loss, and functionality. What influence the right versus the left lobe played in the natural progress of the disease. What the end stage actually looks like: mute, unknowing, profoundly impaired.

Dr. Black was not opposed to MAiD for Sheila, she said. I started to sigh with relief. *But*, she continued, she was not convinced that Sheila could even pass a capacity and consent board hearing. (More on that in a minute.) Dr. Black proposed going with Sheila to the hearing to fill in the gaps in her words. I thought, but did not say, that the capacity and consent board members were in for a daunting, educational day.

Dr. Black sprang into action, arranging for assessments and tests and scheduling the board hearing. Alan sent me regular email updates. The test results were "very discouraging," he wrote. Sheila was in "a turmoil of despair." Meanwhile, Lisa called me, angry: I was to have no further contact with her mother. I assured her that Dr. Black was in charge now, and she rang off, relieved. I was relieved, too. Things were out of my hands. I had to just hope for the best.

In May, four months after my first meeting Sheila and her family, I heard from Alan: he and Sheila had gone to the Stratford Festival to see *H.M.S. Pinafore*. Walking out of the theatre, he'd asked her how she'd liked it. She didn't know she'd been there. The next morning, they sat down and talked. He wanted to retire and travel more. Sheila was spending most of her days sitting alone in the condo. Her children weren't helping him enough, and his own health was being compromised. He felt trapped. He suggested that a retirement home might provide more stimulation for her. She agreed. Alan wrote a long letter to Lisa and Brahm, explaining this. To Lisa, it sounded like Alan was abandoning Sheila when she needed him most. He put their condo up for sale.

"More disruption," I worried to myself, "and time is running out."

In June, Sheila's driver's licence was revoked—a major loss for her. By August, Sheila's children and Alan were accusing each other of stealing from her. It was a mess. I heard Sheila's window of opportunity slam shut.

Cognitive decline is such a conundrum for MAiD, even under 2021's updated laws. If you're well enough to consent to an assisted death, you're probably not ready to die. When you are ready to die, your capacity to understand what is about to transpire may be long gone. Yet it is the touchstone of what I hear most commonly from patients and contemporaries alike: if I'm not me anymore, why am I here?

To determine eligibility back in 2016, MAiD providers used something adapted from the *Tool on Consent and Capacity: Ontario Edition 2003*. The assessor looks at two constructs: the patient's ability to understand and to appreciate. Understanding involves demonstrating factual knowledge about one's condition, including the benefits, risks, and alternatives to treatments as well as an assisted death. Further, it requires that a patient is able to demonstrate some reasoning for requesting help to die. Appreciating involves a realistic appraisal of the outcome of the request—they will die—and some validation of that choice (for example, it's in keeping with their values and beliefs).

In the end, Dr. Black did not think Sheila would be able to convince the board that she could demonstrate her reasoning for her request. Plus, amidst all the ifs and maybes, one truth was undeniable: Lisa did not want Sheila to have MAiD, and Sheila wasn't going to go against Lisa's wishes. I had reached an impasse I couldn't see a way around. I had my practice to run and other MAiD patients whose deaths I could assist. So I stood down. Sheila remained at the back of my mind, though. Her wish had spoken to me.

In 2021, I reconnected with Lisa. "If my mum could see herself now, she would not want to be here," Lisa said. "My brother and I know that emphatically."

Sheila had spiralled downhill faster than even Dr. Black anticipated, in three-month increments. She would sneak out for walks and get lost on her way back. She needed caregivers twenty-four hours a day; sometimes she lashed out at them. She had to be locked in her bedroom at night; she'd bang on the door for hours. She had to be moved several times, from Lisa's home to an apartment to an assisted-living facility.

Lisa quit her job as a kindergarten teacher to care for Sheila. Once, before marijuana was legalized in Ontario, Lisa even drove her white minivan to a boarded-up house to buy a bag for her mother. She hoped it would ease her anxiety. It didn't. Sheila began refusing care, refusing to get dressed.

"Now she has a lot to say, but nothing that makes sense," Lisa said. "Her words aren't real words. She can't even say yes or no. I don't know if she knows me. She can't appreciate anybody or anything. I think she may have cohesive ideas, but she can't express them. So often when I visit her, and I visit a lot, she's just crying." Here Lisa's own voice choked with tears. "I think in a lot of those moments, she's wishing she wasn't here."

In mid-2019, Lisa had contacted Dr. Black about MAiD, but the doctor said no one would do it, not even in Europe. Sheila couldn't consent. It was too late.

"Brahm and I know that in a certain sense, we're failing our mother," Lisa said. "But if we had the chance to go back, even knowing what we know now, we still would make the same decision. She had to be at zero quality of life before we'd consider it. And she wasn't there then." Advance requests, already now law in Quebec as of June 2023, will spell out exactly what that zero quality of life is.

"I will tell you this," Lisa said, just before we said goodbye. "For the most part, this is not my mother. My mother is not alive. I mourn for her. This is a person I love and take care of, but she's not my mum." Even though Sheila is now in long term care placement, Lisa provides for a companion to sit with her mother during all of her waking hours, all day, every day.

I'm grateful to Sheila for connecting me with Dr. Black. Her support gave me immense reassurance when I really needed it. Her burden of expertise is much greater than mine, I think. Most of my patients, including the MAiD candidates, are clear-eyed about their fates. She sees the terror of anticipated decline in so many of hers, and she keeps watch with intimate, in-depth knowledge as they move to the endpoint of these terrible diseases.

As I said, with Sheila, I stood down. I continued on. Her unanswered request, and her ending up exactly where she had so feared she would, became an amorphous weight I carried. It would be added to over the years by other patients I felt I had let down. I would feel that weight from time to time and then shrug it off. Until I couldn't.

CHAPTER SEVEN

Thor

There were too damn many new cottagers around Fenelon Falls, and the road he thought was a dead end wasn't one anymore. That's the joke Thor would make after he'd recovered. But on July 31, 2016, when he told his two adult daughters that he was going for a drive, his purpose had been deadly serious. In the car was a bottle of cognac ("liquid courage"), a note for the police, and a utility knife.

Thorben Jensen was eighty then and distinguished-looking—six foot two, long-legged, and trim with a full head of hair—as well as intelligent, witty, and wry. He'd been living with a rare form of muscular dystrophy for thirty years. When he was first diagnosed, his only symptom was a generalized weakening in his ability to walk. Even then, he often told his daughters, "When it's my time, I'm going. I don't want to be in diapers."

Over the last five years, his symptoms had grown considerably worse. First, he needed a cane, then a second cane, then a walker. He threaded the canes through the walker, too, so they stuck out at awkward angles, because he needed them to ease in and out of chairs.

I say *ease*, but there was nothing easy about it. To rise from a sofa, Thor would first lift each leg into position directly in front of his body and under his torso. Then he would start to rock his upper body forward and backward, while leaning on his arms. It often took him four tries to propel himself out, and he would still be bent forward. To stand upright, he'd have to walk his hands, one by one, up his upper thighs. Then he'd use the canes to manage the gap between sofa and walker.

For Thor, this was unacceptable. He would not be infirm; he'd been fit, hale, independent, and strong-minded his whole life. At age sixty-five, he'd built a stone patio with his twelve-year-old grandson, hefting hundred-pound slabs. Well into his seventies, he'd work for six straight hours in his one-acre garden, then head off for a hike in the woods. He made one concession to his disease: when he had to fell a tree, he'd hire someone to help him—with one condition. If he fell over, which he sometimes did, the helper would allow him time to get up by himself.

The second of six children, Thor was raised in Huntsville, a small town in the Muskokas, a couple of hours north of

Toronto; forests and lakes were his backyard. The only one of his siblings to go to university (Queen's), he studied hard, but he also loved pranks. When a Russian football team visited, he stole their flag; he once "borrowed" a trophy from a police department and dropped it off at a post office. The antics continued into adulthood, too: one Thanksgiving, both his daughters brought home new boyfriends. Karen's had a pierced ear; Kim's was a football player. Thor came to the table wearing dangly clip-on rhinestone earrings with black football smudges under his eyes. He said he wanted to make each young man feel welcome.

Thor began his career as a mining engineer, then became a chartered financial analyst. He started his own business, doing debt-equity financing for mines, and ran it for thirty years, travelling the world. A lifelong outdoorsman, he took regular hunting and fishing trips with groups of friends, sleeping rough in lean-tos. His cottage was full of rocks he'd haul home from his work excursions, and each one had a story. When his clients opened gold mines in South America, he slept in the jungle. To enter a Pennsylvania coal mine, he folded himself in half to ride a conveyer belt through narrow passages. Once on an ice road in northern Canada, he faced a decision: if you drive out today, the road might hold. *Might*. But if you don't, you're here for a month. He took the ride—with all the doors open, so he and the driver could jump free if the truck broke through the ice.

During the last eight years of his career, Thor carpooled to work with Karen, who worked in a downtown tower. His day ended before hers, so he'd sit in her lobby, read the newspaper, and chat with all who passed by. "He knew everyone, and everyone loved him," she told me. He often remarked to his daughters that the worst day of his life was in 2013, when he realized he could no longer navigate his office building.

Thor was seventy when he and his wife divorced, after a forty-seven-year marriage that had grown increasingly troubled. He began seeing Sharon, the widow of his old friend Herb, whom Thor had helped nurse as he was dying from cancer. Thor moved into Sharon's house in Owen Sound, and they spent a happy decade joining clubs and travelling to Florida with friends. But when his disease progressed past the point where he could "properly" be in a relationship, he ended things and moved out. He refused to burden her. He moved into his cottage and installed a lift in the bathroom so he could get himself into the shower.

When Thor retired in 2013, assisted death was not yet legal in Canada. He began researching countries where it was, focusing on Switzerland. He followed the *Carter v. Canada* case closely, and he first asked his doctor for MAiD in November 2015, before the legislation had even passed. When it passed in March 2016, he asked again; when it came into effect in June 2016, he asked a third time. He was adamant: he wanted "the pill." But each time, Thor's doctor declined, because Thor didn't meet the RFND requirement. His natural death was not reasonably foreseeable.

Thor was nothing if not determined. First—at the age of eighty-one—he tried to find a drug dealer who would sell him a fatal dose of fentanyl. When that failed, he began to invite friends to visit him. "It was a very busy time," he later said to me, with a sly smile. Unbeknownst to his pals, he was saying goodbye. He'd planned his "D-Day," the day he would end his life. If no one would give him "the pill," he'd do it himself. On the last day of July 2016, he drove to what had once been a remote area, fortified himself with cognac, and slashed his right wrist with a knife.

Thor's plan had a glitch, however—it was the Sunday of a summer long weekend; cottage country was in full swing. A concerned passerby called the Ontario Provincial Police, who took him to hospital. A nurse there asked him, "How did this happen?" His dry reply: "In the usual way." He left with four stitches and a prescription for antidepressants. Kim and Karen made him promise not to do that again, and to agree to move into an assisted-living facility. In exchange, they promised to find someone who would assist his death. Eventually, they found me.

I'm surprised how long it took me to realize that suicide attempts and MAiD requests were often intricately linked.

In those early days of MAiD, I was preoccupied with doing assessments and approving patients, and the frequency with which their stories included attempted suicide didn't register. But as I went through my notes for this book, I added them up. Well over 60 percent of the MAiD patients I encountered in those first five years had tried (before MAiD was legal) to end their own lives.

In my and my fellow doctors' defence, the warning signs can be subtle in these patients. Many have endured chronic states of disability for so long that the intensity of their suffering isn't readily apparent. Or they don't complain enough to cause *me* discomfort, to question if I can do more: Can I lend my encouragement or boost their flagging morale? Can I find more support workers to help keep them active and connected? Often their physical limitations and their fixed routines mask an inexorable decline in their spirit or interest. It appears they will go on and on, doing less and less, and be okay with that.

Certainly, the elderly patient who booked the guest room in her retirement residence and took an overdose of her insulin shocked her family doctor, who thought she knew her patient well. But prior to that dramatic assertion, had anyone in her family known about her desperation and resolute determination to end her life? How do we determine when they have decided that enough is enough, that they have no more reason to carry on in pain or unable to do the things that bring enjoyment to a day or value to their life?

I firmly believe that for many people, knowing you can have help to die relieves the fear of an isolated, ignoble, or frightening end. Even if they ultimately don't choose MAiD, they know it's there, a brace against despair, a tool of agency, mastery, and even, oddly, hope. Suicide is a furtive, mostly desperate act that someone undertakes alone from a place of defeat or rage. Many patients admitted to me that the thing that stopped them from trying suicide was not dying, but the fear that they would "botch it" and wake up in an even worse condition. For them, a medically assisted death—acknowledged, open, approved, and, most important, supported—becomes the final piece of their lifelong medical care, a rationally made and carefully vetted choice with a safe, painless, predictable outcome. Done well, MAiD is an act of comfort and love.

It's important to note that helping anyone take their life outside MAiD remains a criminal offence. Although Bill C-14 amended the Criminal Code to allow practitioners like me to assist patients who are seeking to die, on their own terms and in their own manner, strict safeguards are in place to protect vulnerable patients. As I've mentioned, there are four criteria of eligibility, and when I meet with patients to ask them why they want MAiD, the first three are relatively easy to establish: they have a serious illness, disease, or disability; they are in an advanced state of irreversible decline in capability; and those things are causing grievous and irremediable physical or psychological suffering that is intolerable or cannot be relieved in any way that is acceptable to them.

But before the law was amended in 2021 the fourth criterion—that the patient's natural death had to be reasonably foreseeable—well, that one confounded all of us who worked in MAiD. It still does. Though the law has changed, people's feelings haven't. Many struggle to accept their loved one's choice, if they feel they're leaving too soon. Thor is a perfect example.

When Kim and Karen first brought Thor to my office in October 2016, he met the first three criteria, no problem. One, he had muscular dystrophy. Two, after thirty years, his disease was certainly advanced, and nothing could reverse it. Three, given how highly Thor valued fitness and independence, his current state of decline was certainly intolerable for him. He rejected the only other solution— more assistance—outright. He'd rather not bathe than accept help.

When I met him, Thor lived in a retirement home in Toronto, to appease his daughters. (Kim told me that on move-in day, Thor had balked like a four-year-old. "I'm not going, no one can make me," he said. She had to discipline him like a toddler to get him into the car.) His new home gave him elevator access, meals, and the opportunity to mingle with peers. Kim and Karen visited often. He befriended the staff, flirted with the women residents, took walks every day, and greeted the neighbourhood regulars he came to know.

But privately he hated it. Too many residents, whom he referred to as "inmates," were ancient, addled, helpless. "There are people who never leave their rooms, except on the mortuary stretcher," he said. This was not how he saw himself. A slow, painful fade was not how he wanted to go out.

He certainly hadn't lost his ability to reason or his sense of fiscal responsibility. He told me that the federal government should be happy to okay his death: it could stop paying his monthly Old Age Security benefit, and it would save on the looming mountain of medical and care expenses he was sure to need. Thor knew he was lucky; unlike many people who are terrified they will outlive their finances, he had enough money. He was just determined to "get out." He said that over and over.

The statistician in him determined that he'd already lost 70 percent of his capacity. But even with his advanced disease, I could not honestly state that his natural death, as the law read at the time, had "become reasonably foreseeable, taking into account all of [his] medical circumstances, without a prognosis necessarily having been made as to the specific length of time that [he has] remaining." I was legally obliged to deny his request.

Thor was angry, to say the least. His single-minded fierceness, his obdurate bullheadedness in pursuit of his goal intimidated me more than a little bit, and it raised questions in my mind about his mental state. Was he endlessly repeating himself because he was determined, or was that another sign of decline? His daughters were reluctant to leave him alone with me; they said it was because his hearing was failing, and he might not answer my questions properly. But was that masking something else? At that time, I tried to limit my assessments to an hour (I've since amended that), but I knew I needed more time with him.

Why an hour? I had conditioned myself that way. During my first months of MAiD education, when I spent time at Sunnybrook's cancer units and in the community, the doctors I worked under taught me the unofficial, unspoken, but still very real rule of allotted time for consults: assessment, conclusion, and recommendations, all in sixty minutes. There were only so many hours in a day, they reasoned; spending more than that on one patient would shortchange another.

So I trained myself. Say hello. Get the history of the event we were dealing with, the treatments to date, a review of past history, and the medications both in use and tried but abandoned. Get a social history, too, including the supports that were in place in all senses of that word: spiritual resources, family involvement, and community services. Do a physical examination. Outline the symptoms that needed to be addressed, such as pain, breathing, elimination. Explain to patient and family what was wrong and how we would remedy it until the next visit. At minute fifty-nine, say good-bye. No wonder I speak quickly.

I would use all that information to determine the palliative predictive score, or PPS, which, as I mentioned earlier, serves as a road map of a patient's trajectory to death. When I knew a PPS, I could order up more services or modify current ones. The family would know when it was time to consider hospice care or hire more help—or when the time was right to seek MAiD. Despite carefully considering all of this, we doctors often overestimate how close death is for our patients. Study after study underscores this tendency, and it frequently becomes a point of pride for our patients: "The doctor told me I only had three months—and that was six months ago!" As if they held a magic key to cheating death and proving the doctors wrong.

On the other hand, a patient's length of stay in a hospice facility is usually far shorter than the expected twelve weeks—it's often less than ten days. To me, this suggests that the caregiving at home, in the hands of an overburdened family member, goes on longer than it needs to. Often, the need to relieve family caregivers of their burden is under-appreciated. Far too often, spouses and adult children burn through their physical and emotional reserves trying to provide end-of-life care at home.

Again, these were the early days of MAiD; we were building the protocols as we went along. But the format I'd learned for palliative care patient assessments became my template for MAiD assessments. For the most part, it worked well.

With Thor, however, I hit a dead end. I simply could not predict, after he had lived for thirty years with his dystrophy, how long it would be before he was completely dependent. I asked him to return for a Montreal Cognitive Assessment (MoCA) test, which I'd also given to Sheila. Doing the MoCA would give me more time with Thor, to get a better sense of his rationale for seeking this end for himself. I needed to get past his rigid insistence and grasp the values that were underneath them.

Thor scored twenty-six out of thirty, almost normal range. It was what I had expected, but I wanted to set a baseline for his reasoning and memory, in case we needed to show that he was declining over time. Somehow, I knew I was in for the long haul with him. As a next step, I set him and his daughters a task.

I gave them a contact number for the British Columbia Civil Liberties Association (BCCLA), which was in the process of mounting a court challenge to the RFND clause. That clause, their argument ran, denied people like Thor their rights to life, liberty, and security of person under the Canadian Charter of Rights and Freedoms.

Already in 1993 the Supreme Court had ruled that "the principle of sanctity of life is no longer seen to require that all human life be preserved at all costs." As for liberty and security of person, in 2015 the court had ruled, "An individual's response to a grievous and irremediable medical condition is a matter critical to their dignity and autonomy. The law allows people in this situation to request palliative sedation, refuse artificial nutrition and hydration, or request the removal of life-sustaining medical equipment, but denies them the right to request a physician's assistance in dying. This interferes with their ability to make decisions concerning their bodily integrity and medical care and thus trenches on liberty."

They were fine words, but they weren't actionable at that time because of the restrictions imposed by the RFND requirement. Before that clause was modified, many patients who weren't actively dying had to endure years of pain and suffering.

I warned the Jensens that the case would take two or three years to move through the courts. But there was strength in numbers; they could add their names. I also reassured them that, though I didn't find Thor eligible now, there would come a day when his death would be reasonably foreseeable. I would keep his file open. When someone comes to me, as I've said, I stay with them until the end.

———

It was now November 2016. MAiD assessors and providers across the country had been working for five months, helping hundreds of people, and demand was steadily increasing. But each case posed its own questions, and those questions were multiplying. Yet each MAiD worker struggled alone to answer them.

Medical professionals are accustomed to operating under clear guidelines. For a family physician like me, the College of Family Physicians of Canada is there to outline what's expected of us, what the pillars of care are. But MAiD brought together a vast cross-population of specialists— family doctors, palliative care doctors, anesthesiologists, neurologists, internists. And no one was issuing workable guidelines for us, not Health Canada, not the regulatory bodies, not the federal or provincial politicians. Not the legal system. We needed working guidelines that we could adopt across the breadth of Canada to address the thorny issues. Coming to a coherent and comprehensive set of such guidelines was an enormous task, one that felt impossible. I was beginning to despair that it would ever happen.

Luckily for everyone—and I cannot stress that word *everyone* enough—a group of doctors in British Columbia, led by Stefanie Green, saw this need and kick-started a grassroots organization dedicated to educating Canadian assessors and providers, while enabling us to connect with one another.

Before Bill C-14 passed in June 2016, Dr. Green was doing much the same thing I was: she was engaged in her own self-administered crash course in assisted dying. In May 2016, she attended a conference of the World Federation of Right to Die Societies in Amsterdam. These four-day conventions, held every two years since 1976 in different cities around the world, are attended by scholars, administrators, clinicians, and do-it-yourself laypeople. At the opening reception, Dr. Green joined forces with five other Canadians: four doctors (Konia Trouton, Jesse Pewarchuk, Ellen Wiebe, and Grace Park, all from B.C.) and an administrator (Darren Kopetsky). They divvied up the lectures, so they could learn as much as possible, and shared their notes.

Once home, they started an email exchange and invited others to join. Two doctors from Vancouver Island signed on, Jonathan Reggler and Tanja Daws. Then two from Nova Scotia. Then I joined, with three colleagues from Ontario. (I glommed onto the thread like glue. I had so many questions.) By summer's end, there were twenty-five of us, sharing information. At first our exchanges were mostly practical:

"Where can I get IV tubing?"

"What IV access point do you use?"

"I think I'll start two lines, because I had one collapse."

"Oh, I disagree. I think two lines is hard on the patient."

"Make sure you speak to your pharmacist; you'll need to have a steady provider for the drugs."

"How do I find a willing nurse?"

"What do you take in your kit on the day?"

"Be sure to contact a funeral home before you do a provision, because the funeral home I called doesn't believe in MAiD. They wouldn't pick up the body."

"Here in British Columbia the paperwork is seventeen pages. What do you have in Quebec?"

"Does anyone know any MAiD providers in southern Ontario? I've had three requests this week, and I don't have time."

"In Amsterdam, they told us self-care was important—maybe take a day off after your first provision?"

And so on.

Soon I was getting scores of emails a week. It was immeasurably valuable, because who else could we ask? Nobody. We could unload to our spouses and friends, but they couldn't answer our questions. We had only each other.

As everyone in the group performed more provisions, the emails grew more personal. We shared moving things that family members said to us; we expressed surprise by some turns of events; we confessed how we felt when leaving a patient's home. We talked about whether we were scared, whether we should keep in touch with family members with whom we'd bonded. Our exchanges are private—almost sacred, really—so I have to keep these details vague. But we weren't engaged in right-or-wrong moral debates. We all chose this work because we believe in it. The sentiments were not, "I don't know if I can do this; I can't follow through." They tended more toward, "I was nervous, but it felt right. I've treated Joe for years, I was glad to be there for him. I'm touched how grateful the family was."

The information was practical, process-driven, full of engagement and debate. It filled my inbox. I would drift off to sleep scrolling through the details of a particularly difficult encounter. Somehow, the macabre humour of some of the encounters drifted through, too, and I would fall asleep smiling.

By the fall, Dr. Green knew we had to become more than just an informal email group. We needed an official organization, not only to issue guidance but to represent the people who do this work. To speak for us and support us. She filed incorporation paperwork and recruited five of her initial comrades to take leading roles as secretary and treasurer and to oversee education, research, and standards. In December 2016, they began working on a conference to be held in June 2017. They put out newsletters. They recruited more MAiD workers. It was all voluntary, and it was nonstop. In March 2017, the incorporation came through. We were now CAMAP, the Canadian Association of MAiD Assessors and Providers.

By early 2022, CAMAP boasted nearly four hundred members, including social workers, lawyers, administrators, care coordinators, nurses, and ethicists. Sixty percent of the members are clinicians, and 80 percent of those are primary care doctors. The organization has produced twelve guidance documents, eight of which have been translated into French. We've held three national conferences. Every six weeks, we hold case-sharing webinars: people review four cases in ninety minutes and share what they've learned.

The initial email chain has grown into three separate online forums. The largest one is for the general membership, where everyone involved in MAiD can meet whenever they want. Then there is a midsized one for those who do assessments, where they can talk more securely and intimately about tricky issues. And the third is exclusively for the doctors who do the provisions, a place where we speak freely with each other about our work, how we feel about it, where the conundrums still lie, and what needs remain to be addressed.

I mentioned that government and the law hadn't developed standards for us, so clinicians had to step into that void and create them for ourselves, based on our experiences. In retrospect, that turned out to be appropriate. It was pointless to look for someone else to guide us, because no one else knew more than we did. We who were providing MAiD had made ourselves the experts. We had to define things very carefully, so we could act with cohesion and comfort. Because if we did it wrong, we faced not only public and professional censure but potentially jail time.

By June 2017, the need to provide clinical practice guidelines for such things as reasonably foreseeable death was paramount. The question "What do *you* think it means?" had been running through our emails for months. "Natural death reasonably foreseeable" is not a medical definition. It's not a legal one, either. A health authority might say, "I think it means three months." A patient might respond, "Hell no, it's three years!" Someone else would say, "It's not about months or years; it's case sensitive."

Eventually, after months of discussions, we determined that *reasonably* should be a clinical decision, meant to be made by a clinician. We worked up a definition; we massaged it. When enough of us agreed, it became the CAMAP guideline. The legal changes of 2021 enforced that our instincts were right.

But in late 2016, when Thor needed an answer, we hadn't yet created our guidelines for RFND. So the question I asked myself was, "How far can I stretch *reasonably*?" I would come to ask that for a lot of patients. My answer was the timeline established by the PPS. In the case of patients like Thor, Ashley, and Yolanda, I had to allow for a trajectory that was measured in years, not months. The *process* of decline, the pain and suffering it caused, both physical and emotional, mattered far more than the timeline.

Still, I knew I would need to justify my long-timeline reasoning to a coroner, who is required to sign off on all MAiD procedures in Ontario. It's a crucial system of oversight, so here's a quick primer on how it works. The coroner's first question is usually, "Tell me about this patient." I begin with the basics: name, address, a brief history of their illness. I'm careful to detail how the eligibility requirements have been met. I mention the second assessor, the date the patient made their request, what drugs I used and in what order.

Then they ask *the* question: "What are you putting as the cause of death?" The cause of death is required on the death certificate. Coroners have a solemn duty to speak for the dead. They must be satisfied with the details I give them, satisfied I got it right. That reassures me; it reminds me I'm not in this alone.

That became even clearer as the popularity of MAiD rose, and coroners began hiring nurse practitioners to handle the volume of these calls. (Last time I checked there were nine in Ontario.) As we got to know each other, they often brought me back into myself, as I told the story of the patient for whom I had just provided. They don't simply jot down details—they're reflective; they share their thoughts about what the patient's life must have been like. Often, I'm moved by a particularly astute observation they share as they hear the story. They bring me back to the emotion of the situation, which I so often put aside in order to do the job.

In Thor's case, I knew I would be giving them a long explanation of why his death was reasonably foreseeable. And to feel comfortable doing that, I needed backup from my fellow providers.

Physicians are more than comfortable when they're providing MAiD for terminally ill people, who are in great pain. If someone is having discomfort in breathing, talking, or eating; if they're cachectic (wasting away), bed-ridden, or in pronounced decline—the decision is easy. With someone like Thor, on the other hand, we assume that he'll find a way to adapt to his compromised circumstances. He'll accept his decline and make the best of it, and we'll provide empathy and counsel. But sometimes our duty of care smashes against a patient's wish to stop it all, to control their own exit from life.

The truth is "grievous and irremediable suffering" is a psychological state too. It's personal. It's an individual's sense of what is intolerable that propels a request for MAiD. It is not me who decides the degree of suffering in a patient. If they say they are suffering, they are. Thor was literally shouting that he was. If he came to me now, I would say yes in a heartbeat. In 2016, with RFND not defined, I had no choice but to say no.

I heard nothing from the Jensens for six months, and then I received an alarming phone call from Kim: Thor had had a stroke while she was driving him from the retirement home to the cottage. She called 911, and EMTs took him to the same hospital where he'd gone after slashing his wrist. He spent three hours in a coma, then slowly came around, confused and shaky. Over the phone, Kim's guilt was audible: Had she done the right thing? Should she *not* have called 911?

I reassured her that, even knowing Thor's wishes, she could not have stood by waiting to see what happened. That is too much for a family member to shoulder in a moment of crisis. She sighed with relief. I also told her that, ironically, Thor's stroke now qualified him for MAiD. I expected she would call for an appointment the moment Thor got home.

I heard nothing. Weeks went by—nothing. Periodically, I asked my secretary, "Have you had any calls from Thor's family?" None.

And then late one Friday afternoon in May came a panicked call from Kim. Thor had fallen and fractured his femur. He was in the ER of a downtown hospital—a Catholic one— and he was ordering the ER staff not to operate on him because he was going to have an assisted death. (His exact

words were "I've been authorized; put me down like a dog.")
He didn't want them to waste money on a surgery.

"That's not how this works," I told Kim. "No one will
leave him lying on a stretcher with a broken leg. You have
to persuade him to let the surgeons do their job. We will
sort out the forms for MAiD after he's out of the OR."
The legally mandated ten-day reflection period between
approval and provision would occur during his post-op
recovery. I also warned her that Catholic hospitals don't
allow MAiD to happen within their walls. We'd figure out
the location soon enough.

Thor's surgery was successful, and he became the darling
of the ward, clear and optimistic in his chosen future. The
surgeons made rounds daily and he greeted them all cheer-
fully, knowing he was going to have his way. Kim took a
leave of absence from her job, and she and Karen spent full
days with Thor, both in the hospital and out for walks with
him in his wheelchair. Karen's son flew in from San Francisco
to say goodbye. For those few weeks, they became regulars
at a nearby brewpub—the owners always found a table for
Thor, in his bathrobe and blanket.

Meanwhile, I was back at Women's College Hospital,
once again convincing the review team to provide space for
an assisted death. The Catholic hospital would discharge
him on the designated day, and Kim and Karen would take
an hour to wheel him north to Women's College. They could

have driven, but Thor wanted one last walk. I would meet him there and help him die.

June 15 was balmy, and the Jensens took their time walking up to Women's College. Thor was even chattier than usual, waving at passersby, making dad jokes about local businesses. ("Hem your pants while you wait? Do they do it while you're wearing them, or do they make you drop your drawers?") At the entrance to the hospital, Kim sat down on a bench and looked Thor in the eye. "Last chance, Dad," she said. "If we go through those doors, you're not coming back."

He replied, "I am so ready."

Me, I was just grateful. Grateful that we had managed to pull this off, despite surgeries, post-op confusion, and another stroke-like event Thor suffered that I haven't even mentioned. Grateful that he recovered fully and was able to consent. Grateful when both daughters told me how happy this last month had been for the whole family. Grateful that, with the end date in his calendar, Thor was elated, positive. Knowing that he would die with dignity and on his own terms freed him and his family to enjoy each other, and to luxuriate in a long goodbye without any pain or fear in it.

Afterward, Kim would tell me that from the get-go, she'd been comfortable with Thor's request for MAiD. "It fit with who he was, intellectually and in temperament," she said. "It's a powerful thing to support someone. And I'm going to say beautiful." Initially, Karen had not felt the same. But over time, as she saw how consistent her father's request was, and how calm it made him, "I had to support him," she said. "It was like saying goodbye to someone going on a trip. Sad but happy, too." In fact, Karen added, Thor's disease is genetic, and she has the predisposition. If she ends up in his position, she'll make the same choice.

I greeted Thor and his daughters in a private room, and we toasted one another with champagne. I explained the procedure, and we began. It still surprised him that it wasn't a pill.

CHAPTER EIGHT

Tom

Thomas Allen Fraser, age sixty-two, had a few character traits in common with Thor. They were both sociable, strong-willed, and certain of what they wanted. But their final chapters could not have been more different.

Tom lived in a one-room apartment in subsidized housing under the hydro towers that run across what used to be northern Toronto, before Toronto spread north of the towers. That apartment had so many locks and instructions posted on his door that it looked like an armed camp. I buzzed. Waited. Buzzed again. A solid click, and the heavy metal door swung open.

I stepped into the room—well, I side-stepped. It was crammed, floor to ceiling, with . . . stuff. Stacked plastic bins full of plastic baggies full of plastic bread-bag tabs, elastics, and matchbooks. Music equipment, including three Sony Walkmans, one in its original package. A vintage

Singer sewing machine that once belonged to his mother. Mounds of cassette tapes (he couldn't afford to buy many CDs, so he'd tape-record the hard rock and heavy metal he loved). Boxes of wires, boxes of mechanical contraptions, boxes of clothes, and cartons of Ensure, the high-calorie, high-protein drink that comprised most of his diet. The walls were decked with motorcycle posters and photos of the Ontario farm where he grew up. It wasn't junk, exactly; there was a sense of order and purpose. But it was a lot. An aquarium bubbled against one wall. A lone chesterfield sat against another.

"In here," a voice commanded. "I'm in bed, and make sure the door is closed behind you." The door had clanged shut, but I dutifully checked it anyway.

A narrow path through the boxes led off to my right. And there was Tom. He managed life from his hospital bed, remotely. He'd admitted me to his flat with one of the many devices he'd rigged. A Hoyer lift—that bar contraption you see in movies when patients are immobilized—helped him access the wheelchair beside him. Which was, by the way, the only seat in the room. This small alcove was as packed as the front room with albums, tapes, radio equipment. More Harley-Davidson posters and photos covered every inch of wall space. Tom was sitting upright. He gazed at me with penetrating blue eyes as I searched in vain for a chair. I settled in his wheelchair.

"You called the ministry requesting help to die?" I asked.

"Give me that file," he barked, pointing to a binder at the foot of his bed. "I am in terrible pain." He handed me a sheet with a highly coloured drawing of a body, front and back.

I was familiar with this drawing. Pain clinics use it as a tool to graphically outline where and how much a patient hurts. On Tom's, the entire back side of the figure, from buttocks to toes, was marked in bright red. The same with both upper arms, shoulders, and the back of the neck. He had labelled the red as "continuous and extreme." The front of the body below the waist was coloured pink and marked "different, lighter pain." He'd written a title on the sheet, "Neuropathic Pain," and had noted in red, "Past seven days—very extreme—pinpoint pins and needles."

"Do you know what a syrinx is?" he asked sharply. "That's what I've got. And I've hit a brick wall."

I did know: a syrinx is a fluid-filled cyst in the spinal cord. The one Tom had was complicated by arachno-syringomyelia, an inflammation of the sheath that surrounds the nerves that come out of the spinal cord and go into the legs. The result is endless pain.

I would soon realize that Tom was in another kind of a pain, too—that of extreme loneliness. He'd always been a stubborn guy. He liked things his way. He'd never married or had children. He'd been in a wheelchair since he was twenty-eight. Because of all that, plus busyness, plus distance, over the years most of his friends and family members had fallen away.

I am used to seeing this grim reality, this unfolding of isolation and shrinking of connections, in the elderly I assess. Friends have died, children have moved away or stopped visiting, too caught up in their own lives. Tom wasn't elderly. Yet he had been hit particularly hard with losses. Did that leave him too much time to be preoccupied by—submerged in—his agony? Doctors were doing their best to manage his pain. But for his loneliness—his extreme aloneness—there was no easy remedy.

Tom was born with spina bifida (Latin for "split spine"), which means his spinal column and cord didn't form properly in the womb. He endured his first back operation when he was mere weeks old, then another at age two. He grew up on an Ontario farm, with a father who believed in pushing his equipment until it fell apart. One of Tom's first chores was to ride the tractor with his dad and pour bucket after bucket of water into the steaming, leaking radiator. It made him competent, though, and frugal. Clearly, he didn't like throwing things away.

Young Tom walked crookedly, wore a lift in one shoe, and struggled with his coordination. Some kids made fun of him, but he had a good pal, Bill, who didn't care about that. Their mothers were friends; the boys went to Sunday school together and ate dinner at each other's houses and played G.I. Joes. (But only at Tom's house. Bill's mom thought they were too violent.) "I was a strong farm boy," Bill told me. "My mum used to say, 'Be careful rough-housing with Tom; you can hurt him.' But he always had a smile on his face. He loved practical jokes. And he had the coolest toys."

When Tom was fifteen, surgeons inserted two thirteen-inch rods in his back to fix the curvature in his spine. It caused a lot of internal scarring and later led to his developing fibromyalgia. When he was in high school, his mother died suddenly of a heart attack, and his dad remarried pretty quickly to a woman Tom did not like. Tom's dad sold the farm and moved the family away. (Tom had an older brother, Fred.) Tom bought a tent and fled the new house whenever he could, camping on his own, cooking over an open fire.

He bought a small motorcycle and rode it for as long as he was able. He grew a goatee and wore his hair long, often in a braid that hung down between his shoulder blades. When the family moved again, to a small town on Georgian Bay, Tom got his own apartment. He was an upbeat guy and made friends in his new hometown. People wanted to help him. They found jobs for him that weren't too strenuous or risky. They watched out for him.

When Tom was twenty-five, surgeons removed the rods in his back but had to leave some screws embedded. For a few years, he used a cane. By the time he was twenty-eight, after three more back surgeries, 265 days in hospital, and the development of the syrinx and the arachnoiditis (that inflammation of the nerves), he could no longer walk. The damage was in his thoracic spine, which runs from the base of the neck to the upper abdomen. Along with the paralysis of his legs, he lost bladder and bowel control. To access more services, he moved to northern Toronto, got a wheelchair, and kept his upper body strong. He played wheelchair basketball at a community centre. He loved music, and he would wheel himself down to Ontario Place to attend concerts, then wheel back home, twenty kilometres each way. Almost every Christmas, Bill and his wife, Diane, brought him to their place in Newmarket, where they run a market garden, and Tom would wheel their two kids around on his lap.

On the hot July day when we first met, Tom preened as he showed me a large map of Toronto, on which he'd outlined in red ink the seven-hundred miles he had clocked one summer in his manual wheelchair. "Boy, you must have worn out a lot of tires," I said. He taught himself to do his own maintenance on everything he owned, even his Hoyer lift.

"It's never good enough, what they give you," he said. "I have to remake everything to work for me."

In his best years, the 1980s and '90s, photos of Tom reveal a buff upper body, shrink-wrapped in a leather Harley-Davidson vest or motorcycle jacket, hair in a braid, bandana on his forehead—the spitting image of a warrior Willie Nelson. In the early '90s, he had a girlfriend, Anne-Marie, who lived in his building and was also in a wheelchair. Tom became her "sort of" lover and a major caregiver for her (she had breast cancer). He cooked for her, took her on outings. They kept their separate apartments, though: Tom needed the space for his stuff, and Anne-Marie's parents did not approve of their relationship. (They were from India, and did not want her to date outside her culture.)

Maybe that's why he wasn't with her when she suffered a seizure in 1993 that put her in hospital. Her breast cancer had spread to her brain. Tom never saw her again: her family wouldn't let him visit her in the hospital, and after she died there, they also forbade him from attending her funeral.

Until then, Tom typically called Bill once or twice a year, to reminisce and catch up. After Anne-Marie died, he began phoning more often. "He was in a low place," Bill said. "More pain. Eating less."

For a few more years, Tom could still lift himself off the floor, as well as in and out of his bathtub and bed. He shopped and cooked for himself. He tinkered. But by 1996, that was over, and the losses of his physical prowess and independence were as devastating as his loss of Anne-Marie. He also had a falling-out with Fred, his brother, and was too proud to reach out to fix it. In 1998, he had an experimental device inserted in his back to stimulate his spine. But it failed, and he had it removed in 2004, amid more pain. And then came more loss: the year before we met, Tom's pastor moved out of town, a friend who sometimes took him out for coffee at Tim Hortons ebbed away, and his family doctor retired. He wasn't fond of his new physician and had seen him only once that year.

As we talked, pain would seize Tom periodically, and he'd fall silent, stiffly waiting it out. At one point, he broke off and grabbed a large container from the shelf next to his bed. "I need my morphine!" he choked out. He spilled pills onto his lap, and I watched with dismay as he swallowed a handful. "Who is managing your pain?" I asked, wondering for a moment if I could do better. But my heart sank as he outlined his regime: high doses of long-acting morphine, a short-acting opiate for breakthrough pain, an antidepressant with collateral effectiveness in chronic pain states. Gabapentin, similarly prescribed for unique pain relief, was meant to ease Tom's burning, bolt-like neuropathy. I knew it was state of the art. I also could see it wasn't enough.

Tom's nurse practitioner, Chelsea Jung, was managing his care. She had referred him to a palliative care doctor who had done two or three home visits. That doctor told Tom that he had "pretty much maxed him out" on pain meds. Five weeks before our meeting, feeling "doped"—perhaps because he'd combined such potent painkillers with a newly prescribed antidepressant—Tom had scalded himself badly, spilling coffee onto his lap. Now he had burn dressings to contend with as well.

In the aftermath of the burn, Tom, like so many of my MAiD patients, had tried suicide—"a lame attempt" with a rope, he told me. One of his personal support workers interrupted him in time and called 911. The palliative care doctor stopped the antidepressant, reduced the morphine dose, and added nabilone, a synthetic cannabis, to his pain-management regime. And now here I was, one last loop for his emotional roller-coaster ride.

Though he was no longer the wheelchair athlete he had been in the '90s, Tom was agile enough as I examined him, lifting and moving his body to accommodate my probing of his wounds. In addition to the burn in his right groin, there were deep friction ulcers on his tailbone and right hip. A wound nurse visited twice weekly to tend to those areas. Personal care workers came by twice daily. Still, Tom told me, he hadn't been out in weeks.

"Loss after loss after loss" went the refrain in my head, along with "increasing isolation over time." I registered his anger, frustration, even desperation. Yet despite all that, my main impression was of a man vitally engaged with living. His boxes of stuff alone were evidence: here was a guy who was determined to be self-sufficient, who wanted to have everything at hand. Who saved stuff, because he might need it, and he might not be able to go back out to get it. He liked his Walkman so he had a backup, in case that one breaks. And the third one, in the package? In case the backup breaks, too. If you're 100 percent determined to die, you don't hang on to stuff.

More importantly, Tom was now phoning Bill almost every night, desperate to recall his younger, stronger self. He would yack away for sixty or ninety minutes—"Remember the time I water-bombed your dad at the cottage in Muskoka?"— and Bill would listen. Bill typically woke up at four thirty a.m. for work; once or twice, he had drifted off as Tom monologued through the evening. "He'd catch me—'Did you just fall asleep on me?'—and we'd laugh," Bill told me later.

Bill would hear the agitation in Tom's voice when the pain got too much. He would keep Tom talking, and "twenty minutes in, I would hear him calming down," Bill said. "He told me the same stories one hundred times, but I had to be there for him. By the time we hung up, he'd be settled down, able to go to sleep. Otherwise, I knew he'd be up half the night popping pills."

Something in Tom's voice made me think I could offer him more than MAiD. "If you could have more pain relief," I asked him, "would you still want to die?

He stared at me. "Of course I'd want to live if I wasn't in so much pain."

"So," I continued, "what if I could arrange a consult for you through the Comprehensive Integrated Pain Program?"

Again, those piercing blue eyes. "I don't really want to die," he said. "I just want to be out of pain."

I had come here to do a routine consult. Did Tom qualify for MAiD? The answer was a resounding yes. The first three boxes were easy to tick off. And his natural death, even at sixty-two, was reasonably foreseeable on many counts: infection, sepsis, accident.

But I'm not much of a box-ticker. I believe strongly in assisted death, of course. But only for people who truly want it. So I called Tom's nurse, Chelsea. I was surprised to learn she had no inkling he had requested MAiD. I called his palliative doctor. Chronic pain management wasn't his area; he was about end-of-life prescribing.

I swallowed. It seemed Tom had acquired another doctor. It seemed it was me.

When you've been in practice for forty-five years, you build a lot of connections that offer back-door channels to consultations, skip-the-line shortcuts. You cultivate them through hallway consultations with your colleagues, phone calls to your old classmates. You ask for favours: "Can you pop in to see this patient; she's just down the hall?" "Can I send you this unfortunate/desperate/deserving person who needs your special approach?"

These asks are becoming rarer: the burgeoning of sub-specialties makes this casual approach impossible. So when I am able to call in these favours, I do so gingerly. Ask your colleagues too often if you can jump the queue, and they stop returning your calls. I also knew that if I couldn't make something happen for Tom, that might well tip the balance for him. It would rubber-stamp his belief in doctors' ineptitude and make him more determined that his only out was death.

I had to act quickly, so I tried two avenues at once. First, I approached my home hospital, Women's College. Several Toronto hospitals had recently amalgamated their various chronic pain programs, which had been scattered across the city, into one comprehensive and integrated academy there. It had the best resources, personnel, and expertise, and because it was centrally run, one referral sufficed. I had already accessed it for another of my patients, and I was impressed with the response. An actual human returned my calls, and she seemed optimistic about the wealth of options they offered.

Second, I called in one of my precious favours and made a connection with a neurosurgeon at Toronto Western Hospital. She had access to Tom's hospital records, because all of his complex surgeries had been done there; it's a centre for advanced research in spinal cord surgery. Was there any surgical intervention that could provide him some relief?

To my surprise, she steered me away from surgery, suggesting instead the Comprehensive Integrated Pain Program at the Toronto Rehabilitation Institute. It functions as an interdisciplinary team that includes specialists in pain management, psychiatry, and orthopedics. The wait time was sixteen months, but she agreed to call in one of her own precious favours to get Tom in.

My gratitude was boundless. I knew Tom couldn't— wouldn't—wait a year and a half. With a huge sigh of relief, I cancelled my referral to the Women's College program and turned all my attention to the Comprehensive Integrated Pain Program. Though the team had access to Tom's records, I bent the ear of the nurse-manager, really driving home the amount of pain he was enduring. I hoped they'd offer him a thorough consultation and a new plan of medication. The stakes were high; the outcome, I felt, was frightfully precarious.

On August 14, 2017, Chelsea called. Tom's opioid use was increasing. Though he consumed a lot of medication, until then he had stuck to the prescribed dosages. He knew if he went over, he'd run out, and he was terrified of that. But now he was taking much more breakthrough morphine, and his mood was dark and low. The pain was unbearable. He wanted help to die. He wanted no more referrals, no more medication adjustments.

Whoa, slow down, said the voice in my head, followed immediately by, I hope I haven't overreached here. I didn't have a Comprehensive Integrated Pain Program appointment lined up yet, but I was certain one was imminent. Chelsea and I agreed on a strategy to reduce Tom's use of breakthrough morphine and increase his synthetic marijuana. We also needed to meet in person with Tom, and we asked his friend Bill (who had his power of attorney for care) to join us at the apartment.

Tom was bleak. His pain was coming in waves, and he was doing what little he could—eating, toileting—"in a rush" before the next attack. "What kind of life is that?" he demanded of us. "I have tried everything. I am done."

Bill looked sorrowful. "This is harmful for Tom," he said. "I wouldn't treat my farm dog like this."

The silence dragged out as three sets of eyes turned to me. I went into calm mode. I assured Tom that he was eligible for assisted death and that I would help him do that. I ran through the details and requirements: he needed to make a formal request before two witnesses who weren't related to him and who would not benefit from his death. (Bill volunteered himself and said his wife, Diane, would drive in, too.) Then there would be a ten-day reflection period, required at that time. I was his first assessor; I would arrange for a second one to come. I outlined the drugs I would use and the route (intravenous) that I'd use to deliver them. I assured him no one would obstruct or decline him.

But, I went on, I have pleaded your case at the highest level, urgently. I am sure they'll respond any minute now. I will arrange a video link, so you won't have to physically get to and sit through a hospital appointment downtown. (In those pre-COVID days, home video conferences were spare and spotty and took a lot of technical arranging, but I was determined.) Chelsea and I would both be on that call. "But, of course, Tom, the choice is yours," I concluded. I did not say, "I am crossing a line here. I am overinvested in you." But I knew it was true.

However, the relief I saw in Tom's face when he agreed to another stab at better pain management made me feel I was justified. I left him with all my contact information, plus a formal request form for medical assistance to die, for reassurance. It was now the end of August.

Recalling the series of debacles that followed can still, to this day, freeze me in my tracks with dismay and regret.

September 1: I receive a fax. The pain program has cancelled the referral, due to a lack of accompanying imaging. I immediately phone the intake nurse and remind her that this is a cross-referral initiated by the spinal surgeon from Toronto Western. I talk her through the details, again. She remembers me; she says she'll obtain the necessary images. Will I be the doctor who signs the agreement for ongoing pain management? (Translation: the pain program will not be responsible for managing Tom's narcotic prescriptions or supervision.) I am not Tom's family doctor, but I'm not about to say no and cause further delays. "Yes," I say. "Send me the contract and I'll sign it."

September 7: The contract arrives. I sign and return it.

September 21: The videoconference is set. We have a two-hour window. Suddenly, the team at Toronto Rehab gets bogged down with an urgent problem. The window is missed.

Chelsea and I scramble to meet with Tom again. She's trying to reschedule the conference link with Toronto Rehab. I'm working with Tom's family doctor to increase his dose of gabapentin. Tom has told his doctor that it gives him some relief, but he needs more. I'm assuring his doctor that I've exceeded the usual three-gram limit with a few other patients, with success. The family doctor is willing. ("Hallelujah" runs the refrain in my head.) We also agree to increase Tom's marijuana dose, again.

While Chelsea and I are with him, Tom moves to hoist himself from his wheelchair into his Hoyer lift, to get back into bed. We try to help him, but we fumble as he is seized by a terrifying bolt of pain. We almost throw him onto the mattress. Exasperated nearly to tears, he yells out, "I have to train you all! None of you know what to do!" We're right beside him, but it's clear to me that he feels horribly alone. He angrily downs a handful of pills.

Then he sighs, a despairing rumble that I can hear in my head to this day. He still wants to live if we can reduce his pain. But he also hands me his signed request for MAiD, witnessed by Bill and Diane.

I am taking notes, furiously jotting down every moment in point form, along two simultaneous threads: one leading to pain management, the other to MAiD. Dread that I have overpromised keeps washing after me. In truth, I have no idea if anything can give Tom the relief he so desperately needs.

What am I doing here? Am I Tom's pain doctor or his MAiD provider? Can I be both? Should I be? This was still early in assisted death, and how involved a MAiD provider should be in the doctoring part of patient assessment wasn't clear-cut. Nor did I have a wealth of previous situations to refer to for guidance.

I'm not his family doctor; I'm not his nurse practitioner. Both of those professionals seem happy to let me charge in with more consultation, more strategies to try. But, *but*, the lines are blurring between carrying the responsibility for the care of this man for living and respecting his request for an assisted death. I am at cross-purposes, juggling two incompatible aims, destined to flounder in both.

Early October: Tom's video appointment with the Comprehensive Integrated Pain Program finally happens, but Chelsea and I are not on the call. Somehow, we have been bypassed in the arrangements. Though I was frustrated at the time, in retrospect, I get it; we weren't vital to the clinic's objectives. Modern medicine is siloed, for better and for worse. The pain program's focus is inward, not directed outward to potential community resources.

On that call, Tom tells them he rates his greatest amount of pain as ten out of ten. He rates his least amount of pain as ten out of ten. Pain interferes with every aspect of his life, 100 percent of the time. They review his medications and note our recent increases. They discuss his wounds, the deep ulcers on his buttocks. Unfortunately, those prevent any additional therapy options, such as water therapy. The only concrete advice they feel able to offer is to try improving his sleep schedule. Tom typically went to bed between two and five a.m. and slept three to six hours. With better, deeper sleep, perhaps he could better manage his pain. They promise to follow up in a month.

Mid-October: The report arrives in my inbox. I am aghast. They have prescribed amitriptyline. Amitriptyline! That drug, an antidepressant, came into prominence in the 1990s as a remedy (unsuccessful, ultimately) for chronic fatigue syndrome. It was a last resort for patients who were felled with such fatigue that getting down the stairs was a major effort. Alarm runs through me. This is the consummate team of pain experts in the largest city in Canada, and a tiny dose of a dated antidepressant is their best answer? Poor Tom, his case is beyond us all, I can't help but think.

I put in an urgent call to Dr. Flannery, head of the pain team. Their one-month follow-up videoconference is in a week. I tell him, "It's imperative that Chelsea and I attend, at Tom's home." In my next unspoken breath, I tell myself, You can't fail Tom again.

Dr. Flannery listens. He understands. But—the same *but* I'd used with Tom, coming back at me—Dr. Flannery is not optimistic that he has any magic tricks capable of shifting Tom's reality. "Pain management in this area is difficult at best," he says. We agree that more opioids wouldn't add much relief. I thank him and email Chelsea, fretting about how Tom is feeling at that minute.

A word about opiates: every Canadian physician is grappling with the opioid addiction crisis. The downward spiral of increasing need and decreasing effectiveness causes a horrifying upswing in addiction and overdose deaths. We doctors have had to confront our own roles in this dismal situation. The targeted, seductive campaign by drug companies advertising "safe" opioid pain management hooked doctors as well as patients. We bought in, and it's more than embarrassing—it's dangerous for our patients and for society in general. Things have only gotten worse since Tom died, but when I was working with him, the knee-jerk solution among doctors when a patient's pain-relief usage was escalating rapidly was to stop prescribing opiates altogether. To cut them off. It didn't make sense. It was a reaction to having been "conned" by Big Pharma, and the result was that many people suffered.

Rules, not need, were defining the duration, quantity, and kind of opiates prescribed. Doctors became skittish about starting patients on any opioids, reverting to over-the-counter standbys such as Advil or Tylenol, even when they knew those drugs would not offer adequate pain control. I had patients who left the ER armed with the advice to take two extra-strength Tylenols, only to call me a few hours later desperate for more potent pain relief. I understood why we doctors let ourselves be seduced: we wanted the best-ever, safest pain relief. But our patients ended up bearing the consequences.

November 3: Tom calls me, irate. His videoconference is today! No one had told him! He has plans for his routine bowel cleanse. Who do all these doctors think they are, weighing in on his treatment strategies, leaving him out of the process? Where were they before while he struggled alone? Doctors are inadequate—"at best," he rails—and not one of us understands or cares about his needs.

"My life," he concludes, "is reduced to getting up to go back to bed. It is not a life." He's wrung out. "I've called Bill," he says. "I'm scheduling MAiD." He cancels the video appointment.

I'm wrung out, too. I call Diane; she confirms that Tom has phoned three times that day to set up his MAiD. We choose a date, November 9. "He wanted to pick a day where we weren't too busy on the farm," she says.

Defeated, guilt-ridden for having created false hope, I arrange for the second assessor. Then, behind on my office schedule, I put Tom "on the shelf" and walk in to see my next patient.

On the morning of November 9, Tom's door swung open for me again. His personal support worker—I'll call her Jane—met me on the threshold. "You do not have to do this," she said, emphasizing every word. She glared at me with blue eyes as fierce as Tom's.

"This isn't about me, or you," I said, as evenly as I could. "It's about choice. Tom has made his."

"I was here all night," she snapped. "I stayed on the couch. He was in his bed, talking on the phone with his niece and nephew for hours. Never once did he take any pain medication. And he was fine, talking all that time, right through the night. We can manage this pain. He does not need to die."

Even his PSW knows I have failed this man, said the voice in my head. I moved into the room and greeted Bill and Diane, who had driven in from Newmarket. They both sported a white rose in their lapel. All three of Tom's regular PSWs were at his bedside, getting him ready.

Fred, Tom's brother, wasn't there. But later I found out that he had visited the day before. "Tom told me not to tell Fred about the MAiD," Bill said. "Tom said, 'He's still mad at me, and I can't even remember why we fought.'" But Bill insisted on calling, and in an hour Fred phoned back. Fred had driven down and was in the lobby, buzzing for Tom, when Tom wheeled in from an errand. "They broke down, hugged each other, and talked for an hour straight, holding hands," Bill said. "It was amazing. My years of listening were all worth it for that moment."

During the years Fred and Tom had been estranged, Tom had missed Fred's kids, his niece and nephew. That's why Tom had been on the phone with them all night—making up for lost time.

Tom's caregivers wheeled him into the living room. He looked fabulous. Radiant. His grey hair was in his trademark long single braid. He wore his black leather Harley-Davidson vest, a white rose of his own in its lapel. He looked joyous. Bill poured everyone a Scotch, neat, and we toasted Tom. (Bill still has the bottle on top of his fridge.) Tom and Bill traded a few last stories, the same old stories—remember the time Tom water-bombed Bill's dad at the cottage in Muskoka? It had been right at dusk, Tom was hiding behind a tree, and bam! Bill had heard the story ten times in the last three days alone. He laughed along anyway. Tom's workers wheeled him back into bed, and we followed.

He turned on his final playlist, culled from his many hard rock albums and cassettes. He sang along. A few songs in, he readjusted the order. He chatted some more. He doesn't want this to end, I thought. I looked around the full room, everyone there for him, smiling at him, and I knew that this was the most connection Tom had had in a long, long time. If he'd had this all along, would it have kept him living?

Instead, he had me. And it was time to begin. I asked for and received Tom's consent. He lay back. He started what was to be his final song, Led Zeppelin's nine-minute opus "Stairway to Heaven." (He was nothing if not a classic, Tom.) I started the midazolam. Anyone who has had surgery, or has even watched a medical show, knows how midazolam works. You begin counting down from ten, and you're usually asleep by six.

Not Tom. Perhaps because he was so accustomed to pain medication—or perhaps because he was so enjoying being with people—the drug was having no effect. Tom was fuelled, energized. "Stairway to Heaven" ended, but Tom was still chatting away. "You're supposed to be asleep by now," I ribbed him. He was prepared for this moment. He reached under his bed and pulled out—a hammer. "Will this work?" he asked, and then grinned like hell when we all laughed.

Eventually, Tom's words became mumbles, and he fell asleep. I administered the last three drugs, noted his time of death, and phoned the coroner. We all waited together in that small, shared space for the call back. I gave my report; the coroner okayed the release of Tom's body. Bill contacted the funeral home. I don't know what happened to the hammer.

In that call to the coroner, the nurse practitioner who answered the line asked, as they always do, "What are you putting as the cause of death on the death certificate?" I had to bite my tongue not to say, "The cause of death is us—our failure to provide social connection, to relieve suffering, to be effective agents of care."

But I knew it would be inappropriate to burden this woman with my felt failure. It couldn't help Tom. I was heartsick that in my stubborn insistence on relieving his pain—the medical solution—I may have missed the point. What if instead I had directed my effort toward relieving the pain of his aloneness—the human solution?

As I stood up to go, Jane, the PSW who had let me in, saw me to the door. "I can see you are upset about this as well," she said, softening. "We were caring for him. He wasn't alone. We could have managed him." Any defensiveness I felt drained away. We met each other's tear-filled eyes.

"I know we will meet again," Jane said. We didn't hug, but I wish we had; we could have offered that small comfort to one another. I have yet to see her again. But I look for her.

Bill and Diane found some solace after Tom's death, through a medium Diane likes to see from time to time. "She said, 'There's someone here in a wheelchair waiting for you,'" Diane told me. "She said, 'He saw you dancing in your living room.'" In fact, Diane and Bill had danced there recently to their wedding song, "Can't Help Falling in Love." The medium told Diane that Tom loved that. She said he had pushed his wheelchair aside, saying, "I'm not in pain anymore."

As for me, by the time Tom died in November 2017, I had been doing this work for almost nineteen months. For the most part, I found it fulfilling. That people should receive help to have a dignified death is embedded in my moral code. I consider it part and parcel of my Hippocratic Oath, to do no harm. If my role with Tom was to see him out, I was fine with that.

But. But before I saw him out, should I have tried harder to bring him back in—into broader company, into the wider world? What if my first conversation had been with his steely PSW rather than his pain management team?

In most areas of my life, I have a surfeit of certitude. I can make big, life-changing decisions in a flash and never look back. But when I am plagued with doubt—oho, that's equally strong. I spend sleepless nights in a froth of What if, who for, why?

Usually I welcome this state of uncertainty. It reminds me that the big questions are unanswerable but need to be asked anyway. I need to think deeply about human frailty. About not knowing. About traipsing merrily down a path, and then realizing it's the wrong one. I believe in a patient's right of choice; I do everything in my power to make sure it's the right choice for them.

But in the end, I'm the one who takes their life away. That is my choice. And I was beginning to feel its consequences.

CHAPTER NINE

Yolanda, Part Two

The first thing I ever noticed about Yolanda Martins was her breathing. It was November 2017, grey and damp. She'd contacted me to do a MAiD consult at the home of her friend Patty, a University of Toronto professor who lived in the Annex neighbourhood, a haven of family homes and small parks. A large oxygen tank compressor loomed on the porch. Yolanda met me at the door, an oxygen tube in her nostrils; extra-long plastic tubing and a rolling tank trailed her everywhere. But she breathed through her mouth, laboured and shallow; I could hear the air moving down her throat. Imagine how you would pant if you'd climbed several flights of steep steps. Now imagine breathing like that all the time.

As Yolanda ushered me into Patty's living room, the effort it took for her to walk twenty metres was so obvious, it felt like we crawled while time stretched. I took in her petite frame, the paleness of her features, the cropped black hair framing her face. It was puffy, a result of steroid medication, I assumed. Her dark eyes were clear and appraising, but the circles under them were deep and almost purple. When Yolanda looked at you, you were seen. No hiding.

So young, I thought.

She fired an opening salvo—"Do you know what LAM is?"—and I understood immediately: let's not mess around. She needed to know what I knew, so she wouldn't have to waste any of her limited breath with the effort of explaining.

LAM, Yolanda would teach me, is lymphangioleiomyomatosis, a rare lung condition. It affects almost exclusively women, literally one in one million, primarily in their childbearing years. Yolanda first had trouble breathing when she was about fifteen. She was forty-five now. For thirty years, hundreds of cysts had grown and crowded together in her lungs until there was almost no room for air. The first time I saw a drawing of LAM, I blanched. The lungs looked like a diseased honeycomb. Grape-like sacs, leaking fluid, where air sacs should be—a wet, oxygen-depriving sponge. My throat constricted just looking at it.

LAM is often misdiagnosed in its early stages as asthma or pulmonary disease. There is no known cause and no cure; the only options are a lung transplant or lifelong oxygen. Without supplemental oxygen, Yolanda's death would be certain, prolonged, and frightening. It would be like drowning or choking, slowly, for three to thirty days.

As she told me her history, I noted how rote and emotionless she sounded. It was obvious she'd delivered this recitation many times. Five years before I met her, she'd had a life-saving lung transplant. In the aftermath, she suffered every complication possible. As with anyone living with donor organs, she was on immunosuppressants, drugs designed to stop her own body from rejecting her new lungs. The hazard with these drugs is that the natural surveillance of the body's immune system to other viruses is compromised.

For example, by adulthood, almost 90 percent of us have persistently infected B lymphocytes from Epstein-Barr virus, a member of the herpes family and one of the most common human viruses. This is countered by our body's cytotoxic T lymphocytes, which basically do a sweep-and-clear function endlessly, so that most of us never even know we have contracted the virus. Yolanda's immunosuppressant drug regimen walloped her T cells and allowed her B cells to proliferate—to the point that she essentially had a cancer of the white blood cells, a leukemia of sorts.

This is relatively common in the aftermath of organ transplantation, but that was absolutely no comfort for Yolanda. She'd been treated with regular chemotherapy and suffered its terrible side effects. She was on prednisone permanently. Finally, newer treatments—biologic drugs specifically developed to interrupt enzyme pathways at the cellular level, and stop the production of her runaway white blood cells—gave her a reprieve. Those drugs increased a patient's life expectancy from six to twenty-four months. Yolanda was now at the end of those two years, and her disease was progressing again in the transplanted lungs.

I could hear her exhaustion. I could also see the formidable person underneath it. I would get flashes of the person she should have been: bright, engaged, adventuresome, with an evident wit. But she'd been forced to conserve her energy for so long, there was no room left for extra anything.

I settled in to listen to her for as long as she wanted to talk—for as long as she could talk—which turned out to be almost two hours.

Yolanda and her younger sister were born in Guyana. Her parents immigrated to Canada when she was five, where they joined a large extended family chockablock with aunties, uncles, and cousins. Her mother was the eldest of nine children, and Yolanda, the eldest cousin; she lost count of how many she had. Growing up in Mississauga, just west of Toronto, she went to Catholic school, took piano and dance lessons, read avidly. Her family took regular vacations and threw noisy parties, where people sang and danced into the wee hours. It wasn't unusual for her mother to cook Christmas dinners for seventy.

Her parents placed a high premium on education: Yolanda had to spend time every summer doing math and reading workbooks. That was fine with her: from age six, she wanted to become a scientist. She studied social psychology, the psychology of group behaviour, at the University of Toronto, where Patty was one of her professors. Later, Yolanda earned a PhD in food neophobia, the fear of new foods, which is often grounded in the mistrust of other cultures.

Yolanda's specialty was crafting questions that would yield full and accurate data. That made her a hot commodity in academia, with her pick of jobs. Because she had always wanted to live in Australia, she chose to teach behavioural science statistics at Flinders University in Adelaide. She was never afraid of big decisions. "If you don't like a job, you leave," she said. "It's like cutting your hair. It grows back."

She loved the work-life balance in Adelaide—no one dared send a work email after five p.m.—and spent her free time hiking, scuba diving, cliff diving, skydiving, and swimming with sharks and manta rays. Looking back, she realized her LAM was in full swing then, but she had attributed her symptoms to other things: breathing too shallowly while diving in deep water, a mild panic attack at high altitude, bronchitis severe enough to have her coughing blood. "Now I know I was putting myself in danger," she said. "I'm lucky I didn't kill myself."

She waited a beat for me to get the joke. Then she continued, "My philosophy was: if I died on an adventure, it would be doing something I loved. I've never believed in waiting to live my life. This is a bit eerie, but my parents tell me that when I was eight, I said, 'I'm not going to live to fifty.' Even before I knew I was ill, I was never able to visualize myself past fifty."

After four years in Adelaide, she wanted to be closer to her parents again. But first she and a friend made a stop in Peru to hike the Inca Trail to Machu Picchu, twenty-six miles at twelve thousand feet. Yolanda could not believe what a struggle it was. She thought she had extreme altitude sickness. She couldn't breathe. She couldn't eat. She had to stop to rest every twenty-five steps. Soon she and her friend had fallen five hours behind their group, and she was chugging coca tea to try to open her lungs. She was thirty-three.

Back in Toronto, dismissed by several doctors as a hypochondriac, she turned to her network of medical pros, who helped her land an appointment at the National Institutes of Health in Maryland. In January 2009, she received her diagnosis: LAM. One of the most severe cases they'd ever seen.

Yolanda was devastated. Though LAM is slow-moving, the median age of survival after diagnosis is only two years. Her doctors estimated she'd already had it for more than fifteen. She was now "tethered to earth"—no more scuba or skydiving. Short plane rides only. For a few months, she cried a lot. She'd recently begun dating a man, and though she was ambivalent about having children, she was sad to lose the choice. She wasn't afraid of dying—she didn't believe in a bucket list, because she'd always done what she wanted to do—but she was afraid of suffering and of the pain her family would feel.

To educate herself, she attended a national LAM patient–doctor conference, and signed up for a series of twenty-minute sessions with experts—everything from the latest research and drug trials to peer mentoring, transplant support, and diet information. She was one of the younger patients there; that was discouraging. But one thing gave her peace of mind: she had friends who, if the time came, promised to help her die. (This was before MAiD was legalized.)

When a job came up at Dana-Farber, a prestigious cancer hospital in Boston, within the Harvard University medical system and with access to LAM specialists, she jumped at it. She and her boyfriend moved to Massachusetts, where she spent five years creating and running data analysis for over a hundred quality-assurance trials. Yolanda loved that job, especially its emphasis on methodology. Researchers would come to her for help to design their studies. She taught them how to hone their methods, "because if you design your study poorly, you don't know what your results mean."

Then she dropped an aside that surprised me. "I purposefully don't read LAM research, though," she said. "I have enough of an identity of my own. I don't want to be defined as 'a LAM patient.' This is not a judgment, but some people get diagnosed and their disease is who they become—they go on marches, they champion their causes. But that's not me. That's not how I want to contribute.

"When you have a serious illness," she continued, "you have to do so much advocating for yourself. You have to decide where to spend your energy. I'm a scientist. I trust my doctors. I understood from the beginning there is no silver bullet."

We'd already been talking for a long time, but I was in no hurry. Yolanda was laying out her data for me, systematically. I could sense she was building to a turning point.

It should have been good news. At age thirty-eight, she was approved for a lung transplant. The operation would be arduous and the aftercare demanding, Yolanda warned her boyfriend, but she was bubbling with excitement at the prospect of regaining her health. That's when he told her he was leaving. It was all too much for him.

In December 2012, Yolanda's mother flew to Pittsburgh, where Yolanda got her new lungs—"stuffed in," because the donor was over six feet tall, while she was only five foot one. As gruelling as the operation was, the aftermath was worse: intractable vomiting, leaks in the new lungs, embolisms, the post-transplant cancerous reaction, kidney trouble. At one point, her weight plummeted to sixty-nine pounds, and she needed to be nourished intravenously by a central venous line. Her mother stayed with her through all of it.

When Yolanda finally accepted that she wouldn't be able to work again, she returned to Canada. She moved in with her parents in Whitby, a small city forty minutes east of Toronto. For her frequent appointments at the University of Toronto's transplant unit, she'd roost here at Patty's. But her life was shrinking. She slept nineteen hours a day. Getting up and dressed was a three-hour process. It took her a year to read Michelle Obama's memoir, *Becoming*; she couldn't manage more than three pages a day. At first, she thought her problem was holding a heavy book, so she got a reading table. Then she realized that concentrating on a page of text wore her out.

Healthy people don't know that being ill is a full-time job, Yolanda said—a job that you pay for, not the reverse. Though she qualified for disability insurance, she had to supply new paperwork every four months to prove she was still disabled. Even with a fatal condition. The drug plan she was on required special paperwork. She spent hours on the phone with insurance providers, being transferred from person to person. Often it reduced her to frustrated tears. Her parents tried to help, but the system was too complex for them. The entire burden fell on her.

Then there was the Wheel-Trans nightmare. Living in Whitby with her parents and no car, Yolanda relied on

Wheel-Trans—a door-to-door van service for people with mobility challenges—to go anywhere. But in 2018, the region introduced accessible buses and revoked her Wheel-Trans privileges. She tried to explain that if she had to get herself to a bus stop, by the time the bus came she'd be too worn out to get on it. They replied that she wasn't "disabled enough" for Wheel-Trans. She had to fundraise to hire a lawyer. She had to get herself to a hearing. Yolanda did win, after three months' work and fifteen thousand dollars in costs. She had recently received a new letter from Wheel-Trans: they were reviewing everyone's privileges again.

On top of all that, she was in constant pain. "They say there's no pain in the lung lining—don't you believe it!" she snapped, in a rare outburst. She found herself a Pilates teacher, a breathing expert who taught her drills to maximize her lung capacity. "If it weren't for Pilates, I'd be dead," she concluded. It made her lung-capacity numbers seem better than they were. For example, her six-minute walk test registered as 40 percent of normal. But she knew that number belied how spent she felt.

Now she was focused on her future, and it looked narrow. Her transplant doctor was one of Canada's best, and a new drug was about to come onto the market. But to qualify, she had to agree to another lung transplant, and that she would not do—because of how she'd suffered after the first one; because it had improved her health for only six months of the past six years; because she couldn't shake the idea that any lungs that would fit her petite chest cavity should go to a child. And because she was exhausted.

"I don't have the stamina or energy to go through it," she said. "I'm worn out."

I was marvelling at the stamina she had in this moment, talking to me at such length. But I also understood what I was seeing: a woman who knew herself through and through, making the case for her death.

"At first the loss is so gradual, you kind of don't notice," Yolanda said. "But for years now, I've felt tired all the time. My lungs don't open and close the way they should, so my muscles are always tight. My body is stiffening because I can't move around freely. I can't get comfortable. My sleep is horrible. Sitting in a chair is work. Projecting my voice is work. I don't like background music anymore because I have to talk over it. It's hard to bend forward because my diaphragm is so tight. I can't make my bed anymore. I can only wear flat shoes. I struggle to follow conversations.

"I don't feel happy. I don't feel depressed. I feel nothing," she continued. "My therapist, who specializes in transplant recipients, says I'm not depressed. It's a normal response for someone who's doing what I'm doing, which is merely existing. Some days all I can do is my one hour of breathing exercises. And if I skip a day, I feel it immediately. I get massages but only to create space between my ribs. I've stopped cooking, which I used to love. I can no longer go out by myself. I'm not getting anything out of my life. I want someone to take care of me all the time, which is very different from the independent person I used to be. I don't feel like me anymore. A long time ago, I promised myself that when I couldn't travel, when I lost interest in it—when I lost interest in participating in the world—that's when I would know it's time.

"It's time," she concluded. "It's time for me to say goodbye. My body has been fighting this disease for more than half my life. I'm ready to stop fighting. I still have moments of happiness, with friends and family. I have moments of sadness. But I'm not angry; I've never been angry. This is my path. I'm going to die from this disease. There's no saving me from it. The only question is Will I have a peaceful death or a terrifying one?"

I wanted to wrap my arms around her. I wanted to weep—for her bruising ordeals; for the potential greatness of her life's work, now abandoned; for the randomness of this cruel disease. Instead, I did what she needed me to do: I assured her that she qualified for assistance to die.

I went over the process and requirements. I suggested that her doctors would want to be there to see her out. I told her that if she were my patient, I certainly would. I gave her all my contact information, just in case. But, I explained, I was not attached to her hospital group, University Health

Network (UHN), in any way. I had no privileges or access. I was as powerless in that machine as she was in mastering her disease. The best I could do was link her with one of my colleagues who did have privileges. I told her not to worry; I was sure her UHN team would feel the same way I did. I was sure they'd take care of her.

The next day, I called my UHN contact and outlined Yolanda's story. I told him I'd approved her request, but the corroborating assessment should come from someone already on her team. He agreed—when she was officially ready, the transplant team would pick this up. They wouldn't need my consult note.

I thought I could leave it at that. But over the next months, I was surprised by how often I'd find myself thinking about Yolanda. Unbidden, that image of LAM-riddled lungs would spring into my mind. I would feel a strong urge to call and find out what had happened to her. But that seemed ghoulish. I had turned her over to her own experts in good faith. She had a mighty will. She understood the system. If she couldn't navigate it, no one could.

Let it go, I told myself.

CHAPTER TEN

On the Brink

I first noticed something was wrong with me on a plane, flying from Toronto to Vancouver in June 2019. I should have been excited. Not only did I have five precious hours to myself to catch up on medical journals, but I was en route to the third conference of the Canadian Association of MAiD Assessors and Providers.

By this time, CAMAP had grown into an essential repository of education, advocacy, support, and research. It filled me with pride, and I valued my participation immensely.

I adore my husband and I rely on him. I have a supportive family and network of friends. But I'm hesitant to talk about my MAiD work even with them, because the questions it raises can seem ghoulish or morbid. If I am assessing a ninety-eight-year-old woman whose friends have died, whose family is largely absent, who has nothing and no one to live for, I can log onto the CAMAP forum and ask the question I couldn't ask anywhere else: Can extreme old age plus loss of social connection equal eligibility for MAiD? (Under the 2021 legislation, the answer is yes, but the answer used to be murky.) Does it cause irremediable suffering? Late into the night, I'd be reading more than a dozen replies to that or any question. Not yes-or-no answers, either—long, considered, nuanced discussions. The information-sharing service had evolved into a pillar of support that I counted on.

So why wasn't I looking forward to face time with these essential colleagues? Mingling with them was much more exhilarating than most of the conferences I'd taken myself off to over the past forty years. Many of those had been obligations for my CME—continuing medical education— and I'd grown comfortable with dozing off if a presentation droned on. But CAMAP conferences buzzed with energy, common purpose, and affirmation. Especially that first one in Victoria in 2017: more than one hundred participants had turned up, and we happily pounced on one another, putting names to faces and continuing in real life the conversations we'd been sharing online for months.

MAiD was a moving target; there was new information all the time. So 2019's conference should have been the highlight of my year: triple the attendance of 2017 (already!), jammed with talks and side sessions, everything from the latest research to hands-on demonstrations to presentations by special interest groups. I'd even convinced Laurie Morrison, a medical colleague who was thinking of becoming a MAiD assessor, to come along. Canada needed more providers, and I hoped that the collective energy and commitment of the pack would entice her to join us.

Then why was I feeling so flat, even anxious? I was carrying a lot of patients, I knew that. Few of them were clear-cut cases; they all came with a kind of weight. One wanted to keep her request for MAiD secret from her family. Another was in chronic pain, but he was only in his fifties. A third was, frankly, difficult; though eligible, she'd changed her mind twice already, both times at the last minute, with everything in place and ready to go. I was beginning to glean that she didn't want to die. Was it attention she craved? Was she just afraid of dying, and could I do anything to assuage that? Was aloneness driving her decision more than suffering?

When someone makes a request, I take it seriously; I know I will be carrying their file open for weeks or months, until the provision occurs. That habit led to a deepening involvement with my patients, maybe deeper than was warranted. It seemed I didn't know where or how to draw the line.

I was dimly aware, too, that I'd begun to dodge new requests. MAiD doctors are famous for responding quickly when someone contacts us—even faster than emergency surgeons, I often joked. But lately I found myself saying to my receptionist, "Take a message, I'll call back." Too often I found myself thinking, Just give me someone who's actually dying.

As well, it was dawning on me that my vision for MAiD—that it should be part of every family doctor's cradle-to-grave buffet of care—was not going to pan out. I had hoped for an algebraic growth in MAiD doctors: a family doctor would refer a patient to me for MAiD; I'd invite them to the provision to show how it's done. I would then offer to support them, as a second assessor, when their next request arose. Then they would provide for their future patients, while teaching other doctors to do the same.

That wasn't happening. Doctors were only too happy to refer their long-time patients to someone like me. They were sometimes willing to attend the provision to support their patient. But learning to do it themselves? No thank you. As a result, 85 percent of Canadian provisions were done by doctors who were strangers to their patients. We spend one hour with them, doing an assessment, and that's it. In other words, people were entrusting their last moments on Earth to a person they did not know and who didn't know them. That did not sit well with me.

I kept a journal of sorts, a record of each patient I provided for. I jotted down in a notebook some biographical details—one page per person, maybe two. From that I'd craft my consult notes: who they were, why they'd made the request, their backstory, an accounting of the values that had brought them to this point of no return. A mere three years in, it was gnawing at me that I was losing their names and stories.

Alarmingly quickly, MAiD was becoming its own specialty, and an elite one at that. We providers were hard to find, tough to book. I didn't like that for patients: the last thing I wanted for people who requested help to die was to make it more difficult. I didn't like it for myself, either. The smaller and more select the group that does MAiD, the more we discuss it and refine it, the more we and we alone are called upon to interpret new legislation, the wider the gap grows between us and everyone else.

It reminded me of a period in my forties when my medical partner, Carolyn Bennett, and I suddenly woke up to the fact that were doing three hundred births a year. I was delivering thirteen babies in a weekend; I was pretty much living in the delivery room. "We are not family doctors anymore— we are GP obstetricians," I said to Carolyn. "And no one is coming in behind us to help." MAiD was now feeling much like that.

Also thrumming away just under my consciousness (where I like to shove things that discomfit me), I'd had my first complication with a coroner. The patient was eighty-two, suffering from interstitial cystitis. It's not a life-threatening illness. She was a bit frail, in constant pain, but I knew I would need to catalogue all her other medical problems. The elephant in the room was the cost of the very expensive retirement residence she was living in—and the prospect of outliving her resources to afford staying there. Which meant a move to one of Ontario's public long-term care homes.

I hadn't asked her directly if this was the reason for her MAiD request. I'd learned to ferret out the answer to such questions in the details of a patient's life and work. I knew from my time with the community palliative team how to estimate the costs of care and the escalation of necessary supports to maintain this frail elder in comfort.

But I'd also learned that an alert coroner would quickly piece this together anyway. Coroners are like cops; they see a lot. To the dead, they're defenders; to MAiD providers like myself, they are the arbiters of our actions. Any detectable coercion will disqualify a patient's request for MAiD. This can be financial pressure felt by the patient, who may think their ongoing care is eating into their children's inheritance. Or it can be pressure from family members for the same reason. After my patient died and I explained her situation to the nurse practitioner who answered the coroner's line, there was a long silence. "I have to walk this down the hall," she said.

Ominous words—she wasn't convinced by the explanation I'd given. She had to confer with the coroner. And if the coroner deemed this death suspicious, that would hamper my ability to provide in the future.

There are serious consequences if the coroner decides a doctor's judgement in establishing a patient's eligibility is suspect. At worst, the coroner could deem the act criminal. Or they could report the doctor to their college of physicians, where the doctor may face discipline or suspension of licence. Less awful but still bad, a coroner is likely to be examining that doctor's future provisions extremely closely.

That is why two assessors are required to establish the eligibility of a patient for MAiD and indeed two of us had agreed. But only one of us was there at that moment, justifying our decision about taking this life.

At that moment, all I could do was wait for the call back. I sat with my patient's two daughters for an hour, explaining the glitch, outwardly calm, inwardly stewing. Finally, the phone rang. "You can release the body," the nurse practitioner said. "However, you are on notice." No one ever followed up, which meant the death passed muster. But I was rattled.

Then there was Ed. A patient I'd recently provided for, Ed was the most alone person I had ever encountered. He was in his early sixties, suffering from acute angina and multiple blockages in his heart. Julie Campbell, the intake person who had referred him to me, told me he probably just needed a stent, but the doctors who assessed him had terrified him with the prospect of suddenly dropping dead. The fear of a sudden, uncontrolled death may deservedly drive a request for a planned, controlled exit.

I phoned the emergency cardiologist. Would he please review Ed and reassure him that he can have the surgery safely, and he won't die? A few days later, Ed called me back. He was not reassured. In fact, now he was hurtling toward MAiD. He was giving his pets away; he was driving his cat to Niagara right now; he was terrified that he could die of a heart attack on the road, and what would happen to the cat?

This was feeling like Tom all over again, and I didn't want to make that mistake: I didn't want to become Ed's doctor. I phoned his treating cardiologist (a different doctor from the emergency one I'd asked for reassurance). That backfired. She was outraged. "He's refusing surgery for a remediable condition?" she said. "Then he's a psych case! How can you deem him eligible?" So there I was again: Ed had no one but me.

On the day of Ed's provision, he was alone when I arrived. A young man turned up but only long enough to fetch Ed's shaggy dog, the final pet to be adopted. Ed then Skyped with his brother in England, but the brother signed off before I administered the drugs. When Ed's pastor showed up, I was so relieved I almost hugged him. But after Ed died, as I waited for the coroner to call back, the pastor rose to leave. "The funeral home will come for the body," he said.

"What do I do about the house?" I asked his retreating back.

"Just leave it," he said.

So that's what I did. I sat with Ed's body for the long, slow minutes until the coroner phoned. Then I left and closed the door behind me, hoping the funeral home would come soon, trying not to think of Ed there alone, alone, alone.

Writing this now, it seems obvious that I was headed for a fall. But at the time, it felt like I was hiking up a narrow trail in a dense fog. There was this twist and that turn, and I was navigating blind. I wasn't thinking about the general danger; I was focused on each specific footfall. So when I stepped over the cliff, I was in mid-air before I realized it.

That third CAMAP conference began well enough. André Picard was the keynote speaker. A renowned health reporter for the *Globe and Mail* and the author of *Neglected No More*, an important look at the current state of elder care in Canada, Picard was an early advocate for the legalization of MAiD. I'd heard him speak several times, and I always found myself nodding in agreement. That day, he described how the media's reporting on assisted death was improving: writers were concentrating on the quality of life rather than the quantity of years. Patients were choosing to improve their lives by shortening them, and the result was surprising. In areas of Canada where MAiD was available, the number and quality of palliative care options had improved markedly. I nodded my agreement.

That was good news. People should want MAiD rather than need it. So, as I went into the final lecture of that morning—"MAiD to Last: Creating and Sustaining High-Quality Assisted-Dying Services"—I was feeling okay. A bit cocky, in fact. The speaker, Dr. Andrea Frolic, is many things: a medical ethicist at Hamilton Health Sciences, a social anthropologist, an artist, and a dancer. She and I had talked on the phone two years before, about Ashley, and I had appreciated her listening ear.

But Dr. Frolic is not a medical doctor. She describes herself as a "professional doctor watcher." And it seemed she was going to tell us how to sustain ourselves while providing MAiD. Yawn. Over the previous three years, I'd heard many such talks, and all of them went in one ear and out the other. "Being kind to yourself" was someone else's concern, not mine.

"I'm going to throw a few grenades your way," she announced. I cocked an eyebrow and thought, To this group of seasoned pros? Good luck.

She started throwing: What is suffering, and can we quantify it? How? Who judges? What is competency, if the goal of your treatment is the patient's death? What is exempt from the Criminal Code, and at what point does MAiD become manslaughter? How can a MAiD provider be both a patient's advocate and a participant in her death?

I swallowed. This was not the lulling, reassuring speech I'd anticipated.

"In the Netherlands," Andrea went on, "MAiD is not viewed as normal medicine. In fact, the government gives the doctor a day off after a provision, so she has time to integrate the experience into the fibre of her life. This in a country where the statistics are the exact reverse of Canada: 85 percent of Dutch MAiD deaths are performed by their family doctors. These doctors know their patients. And they do far fewer provisions—the average number might be five per doctor in their career."

Five. I was beginning to feel oddly warm. I had at least five MAiD patients on the go *right now*.

She continued: Dutch doctors admit that every death affects them. And they don't soften the language, either. They don't "provide" for patients. They kill them.

That is a word I do not let myself use.

Suddenly I remembered a conversation I'd had a few months earlier, one I'd dismissed in my usual way. My husband, Bob, had had lunch with a lawyer friend who'd asked, "Is Jean talking to anyone?"

"What do you mean?" Bob asked.

"Well," the lawyer replied, "when any other first responder—a police officer, an EMT, a firefighter—is involved in an active death, where someone doesn't just die but is killed, not only can they speak to a professional about the experience, they must."

At dinner that night, Bob asked me the same question. I looked at him askance. "Well, I debrief my nurses, so they can express how they—"

"No, honey," Bob cut me off. "The doctors."

"Oh, maybe the younger doctors might need to—"

Bob cut me off again. "Jean. I mean you."

"I'm fine, dear. I'm fine."

I shook off that memory and turned my attention back to Dr. Frolic, who had built to her final point: MAiD, she concluded, is "high-risk medicine."

Pardon? I knew high-risk medicine. Trauma is high risk; emergency medicine is high risk. I'd been a family practice obstetrician for thirty years, and there's nothing higher risk than that. An ordinary, dull delivery takes a wrong turn, and in one flat minute you're sweating blood. MAiD was nothing like that. My friends joked darkly that I could never get sued for malpractice—"unless your patient doesn't die, har har."

But Andrea was way ahead of me. MAiD is high-risk medicine, she said, not for the patient. For the doctor. By all estimates, looking at the rising number of MAiD requests and the available providers, we were on track to be short by seven hundred doctors. This was not going to be sustainable.

There's not going to be enough of us, I thought, and it's going to come down to a few others and me. *Me*.

"If you don't take care of yourselves," Frolic said, "the system will fail." MAiD providers will burn out from compassion fatigue, from traumatic grief. From—and this phrase struck a chord—soul collapse.

Rarely do I rush the podium after a speaker wraps, but Dr. Frolic had gotten to me. I wanted to thank her and to remind her that we'd met by phone. I waited until all the other doctors mobbing around her had concluded their chatting and hand-shaking. Finally alone, looking into her welcoming face, I began, "I just want to say that your talk—"

To my horror, my throat closed. My voice seized. My eyes filled with tears. Andrea looked at me, her puzzlement softening to compassion. I was mortified, dissolving in front of her, the epitome of the thing she'd just warned us about. Soul, collapsed.

She began to say, "We should talk," but I was already in full flight—out of the conference room, out of the hotel, down the long walkway to Vancouver's waterfront. My mind was a blank; my feet, a blur. I don't know how long I stood looking out onto the ocean. I only knew that I felt raw and profoundly shaken.

How could I face Laurie Morrison, whom I'd hoped to recruit? (Luckily, she'd found a group of anaesthetist providers and was having a fine time.) How could I face my colleagues, who would surely feel my betrayal?

That's how I thought of it then—as a betrayal. Things are different now; CAMAP has become a forum where providers express their doubts and anxieties, as well as share essential information. But in those early days, we had to be cheerleaders for one another and for MAiD itself. At that conference, there was little room for expressions of doubt. We all shared a tacit understanding that we had to get farther down the road to general acceptance before we ourselves could admit frailty.

In that moment, my frailty felt like moral failure.

I was deeply invested in and committed to this work. But suddenly I could see a future—a very near future—where it ate up my reserves. I'd always felt them to be boundless. I was the person who could deliver babies for forty-eight hours straight without sleeping. I was the person who could narrow her focus in a MAiD procedure down to those seven syringes. If I was breakable, who was I?

After one last shuddering sigh, I willed myself to go back inside. The next meetings would address an issue vital to me and to all MAiD providers: defining guidelines for assessing patients with cognitive issues. We needed a solid platform of agreement for assessors, to troubleshoot declining cognition in patients who were requesting help to die. We had to be able to see them out before they lost capacity to consent on the day. We all had stories about how we had failed a patient, missed the cues, not acted early enough. I should have been first in line, telling Sheila's story. Instead I moved through the rest of the conference mute and numb. At the airport, Andrea Frolic stood a few people ahead of me in the check-in line. I pretended not to see her.

Back home, I tried to shelve the entire episode and get back to work. But memories kept cropping up, needling me. First, I remembered that I'd had a similar collapse once before—years before, when my first marriage was breaking down. I was spending almost all my time then in delivery suites, running from floor to floor at Women's College. I was zooming down a back stairwell, thinking about how to get my kids to their dad's that night, when a certainty washed over me: I'm going to lose it. I ran straight out of the hospital and didn't stop until I hit Queen's Park, two blocks west. I collapsed on a bench, the noise of traffic whirling around me, and I howled.

It was the first time I let myself crumble. I was in the midst of my life, and then suddenly I couldn't be. All the things I had shoved aside to think about later crashed in at once. After about thirty minutes of flagrant sobbing, my inner voice (my father's voice?) said, That's enough. I went back to work.

Second, I remembered my first experience with a person who'd burned out. It was early in my practice. A young patient who worked in a women's shelter—a sensitive, idealistic advocate—came to see me about getting time off. She was helping to take care of her brother, who lived with significant deficits from cerebral palsy, caused by a birth injury. She'd taught him to use a bliss board as a tool for communication, and he had blossomed into a published poet. But recently, an irate husband of one of the shelter's residents had been terrorizing the place. He'd disturbed my patient so much, she was unable to go back to work—literally unable to get herself across the door jamb.

I okayed her medical leave, though at the time there was little compassion for or understanding of traumatic stress disorders. (Those were the days of unemployment insurance and mental illness, not Ontario Works and mental health.) But as weeks turned into months, and my patient continued to shed tears in my office, it was clear to me that she did not have it in her to return to her job. I encouraged her to look elsewhere for work. I still don't know if that was the right solution—did I encourage her victimhood to dictate her life?—and her burnout carved itself in my mind. Can a person lose the will, not to mention the ability, to persist in a vocation that takes everything she's got, yet gives back too little in return? Was that person now me?

Third, I kept thinking about the metaphor for resiliency that Dr. Frolic had used in her talk: a backpack. She even pulled out a real one, which she placed on the lectern in front of her and unpacked, showing us things that meant something to her, that sustained her. A seashell with a hole in it, a gift from her son. A scarf. A painting. Pre-meltdown, I'd found it hokey. Though I did like the seashell, flawed but perfect, because it was a gift from the heart. I tried rejecting the backpack idea, but it ended up saving me. (My father used to say, "For someone who is supposed to be so smart, you can be awfully dumb." He was knocking on my door.)

It took three weeks for me to realize that the sense of dread I had felt in Vancouver had left me. Gradually, I realized I wasn't avoiding MAiD calls and texts anymore. I was willing to consider what would sustain me. Where would I look if my soul was seeking solace?

The first prod came from one of my own patients, Liz. She was about to leave for a year in Germany, and while there, she planned to write a book about surviving middle age—and, she said casually, her metaphor was going to be a backpack. I laughed outright, then found myself yammering to explain why: conference, Frolic, backpack, shell. Then in a gush of embarrassing words, I told Liz what I'd barely told myself. "It was me who had the broken shell! Frolic poked me and the whole facade collapsed!" I thoroughly hijacked Liz's appointment, something I'd never done before. Afterward, I was shocked to look at the clock—I'd disgorged for twenty-five minutes.

The second prod came from a MAiD patient whose provision was two weeks away. She told me she was preparing "little packs" for her friends as mementos of her, filled with tokens and keepsakes of their shared tears and joy. Each included a packet of seeds to plant, to sustain her memory long after she was gone. My urge to take up the backpack theme with her was intense, gaspingly so. But unlike with Liz, I gave this patient the gentlest of hugs and left her with her thoughts, not mine.

Back home, I chided myself. How could I have missed such obvious cues? I am the queen of backpacking! I have lived out of backpacks on the Pacific Crest Trail, trekking in Nepal, cruising the continental divide in Montana. I recently moved, and in packing up my house, I discovered no fewer than twenty-seven backpacks. (I kept six.)

I carry the MAiD drugs to patients' houses in a backpack.

A backpack was even a cornerstone to my marriage. My fiftieth-birthday present to myself had been a three-month hike on the Appalachian Trail, where I hauled a fifty-pound pack over one thousand rocky miles. I first read about that legendary route from Maine to Georgia in my teens, in an issue of *National Geographic*. My dream to tackle at least some of its 2,200 miles lay dormant for years. Suddenly I was forty-nine, shaking off a failed marriage and realizing my three children were almost grown. What better way to stride out of one phase of life and into another?

At the last minute, I invited my newish boyfriend, Bob, to join me, and it turned out to be a bonding experience that transformed him into my second husband. On the trail, Bob and I rarely walked together. Pacing ahead or behind, we each had a lot to digest. He was in recovery for an addiction; I was trying to figure out who I would be now. We'd sleep on the trail for seven days in a row. On the eighth day, out of food and fuel, we'd hike to the road and hitch a ride to the closest town. We'd find a cheap motel, do our laundry, take a blessed shower, make quick calls home (this was pre-cellphone), and restock.

There were challenges, unconscious tests of each other's mettle and staying power. We blew up three stoves. We almost stepped on a rattlesnake in our haste to outrun a thunderstorm. We ran out of water constantly and had to filter litres from mud-holes and stream-trickles. Yet at the end of that journey, there we stood, a newly minted couple.

I'm not tall—that backpack was nearly as large as I am. I'm sure I resembled nothing so much as a snail. But that pack was literally and figuratively a tool kit for resiliency: it held jackknife and stove, food and shelter. It housed the framework for testing my new relationship. It was a challenge to my grit and capability. It gave me freedom and a new independence.

Why was I now running away from this thing I valued? My best character trait is that I don't disclose much of anything to anybody. It's also my worst character flaw. I heard my father again: "You have to be hit over the head with a two-by-four before anything gets your attention."

Damn you, Andrea Frolic, I muttered to myself, you're right. I need your stupid, brilliant backpack. I need to fill it with things to keep me going, to protect me, to sustain me. "They have to be your tools," Andrea had said. "You must craft and create them yourself."

The minute I accepted this, the things I needed appeared almost magically. Part of the art of helping people die is to stay open to new ways to live. Recently, I'd provided MAiD for an elderly Jewish woman. As I was preparing the drugs, her children eulogized her with Jewish prayers. Evocative, blunt, full of truth, they addressed death and loss repeatedly—as laments must. As the words and sobs resounded through the apartment, I was staggered by the force of them. Finally, the mother held up her hand. "No more," she said. She was ready. Her children were ready. It was my time to step in. Afterward, I asked the family to send the prayers to me. They were the first things in my new backpack.

The next item was my version of Andrea's perfectly imperfect shell. As I've mentioned, my dad was a carpenter as well as a farmer, and tools cluttered our basement. When I was ten or eleven, I found a chunk of wood that begged to be carved. With one of my dad's jackknives, I turned out a male figure. The nose wasn't great. The chin was okay. But

I was thrilled with the head, perfectly proportioned, sculpted smooth. You could put your hand on it and feel every knob.

I showed it off to Dad. "What's it about?" he asked. I hadn't thought of that, but I blurted a reply: "All the starving people in the world." I'm still not sure where that came from. But he nodded. It now sits on the hutch in my cottage, where I look at it a lot. It carved itself. It did that for me.

At age seventy, I took up woodworking again, turning bowls and lidded boxes. Most are small enough to be held in one hand, polished to high gleams. I push myself to make them as thin as I can, because that's always a wonder for me, how close you can come to total failure after hours of painstaking work. The wood leads me—a precious change from the rest of my self-directed life—and only after the bowl is finished do I marvel at the unconscious combination of awareness, calibration, concentration, and dedication required to uncover the inevitable in the grain. My favourite is a palm-sized bowl, perfectly turned, but one I'd pushed too far—in my zeal to make the base wafer-thin, it cracked. But, as Leonard Cohen said, that's how the light gets in. That bowl went into my pack.

Speaking of musicians, I recently added two songs to the pack. In the summer of 2020, I helped a seventy-something patient I'll call Fred die in his back garden. The outside venue allowed many more family and friends than would have been legal indoors, because of COVID-19 restrictions. We also did it later in the day than I usually do. Typically, the pharmacist delivers the drugs to my apartment by eight thirty a.m., and I'm en route to a patient by nine. "What's the rush?" Fred had asked me. So by late afternoon, when I arrived, his living wake had been going on for hours, and the garden was a swirl of food, flowers, champagne, and music.

That didn't surprise me. There are no rules for MAiD provisions; families have complete control over the order of service, and many of them turn into tender or raucous celebrations. Fred interrupted the chatter to speak: though he and his girlfriend had been together for seventeen years, they had never gotten around to getting married. But if they'd had a wedding, this would have been the song they danced to. Out poured Louis Armstrong's "What a Wonderful World." I've heard that song hundreds of times—Armstrong's gravelly voice, evoking the extraordinary richness of ordinary life. But as I sat in that backyard, with the afternoon light slanting in, and people swaying, and a breeze that smelled like white flowers, I heard it anew.

I had tears in my eyes—everyone did—but the next song knocked me flat: Dame Vera Lynn crooning "We'll Meet Again." I was a war baby. My sisters' lives and mine were infused with the songs of that era. In fact, Dame Vera had just died, at age 103. I loved how that song floated from generation to generation, binding people together. In that garden, people clustered, COVID be damned, to hold each other close. So I'm holding on to those songs.

Before Dr. Frolic's lecture, I had heard many MAiD providers speak about the rituals they create for themselves and the families they serve to mark the deaths as special. Candles for each family member to light and then blow out, that sort of thing. These rituals never held interest for me, driven as I am to get the job done with efficiency and cool professionalism. For me, it was the family's job to feel complex emotions. My job was simple: maintain the IV lines. Is the flow smooth, are the transitions seamless, is the next drug ready? I lead the ceremony by disappearing from it. I perform but am not really present. I like to stand behind the patient, if I can; the focus is them, not me.

But post–Dr. Frolic, that hokey backpack has become a lifeline for me. I've filled it with meaningful bits of lived experience that have brought me to where I am. It frames my purpose and bolsters my convictions. And it wouldn't be complete without one other thing: poetry.

All my life, I've collected words and images. As a girl, I filled scrapbooks with magazine articles about world events. As a young teen, I found in an old farmhouse behind ours a massive trove of World War II photo journals that kept me occupied for many happy hours. As an adult, I discovered poetry, the ultimate synthesis of words and images, and I tucked poems everywhere: folded into my wallet, stuffed into a drawer at work.

Now I have a notebook, which my nurses put together for me when I stopped doing obstetrics. They filled the first ten pages with notes and messages for me. I have begun filling the rest with quotes and poems. The end of one phase, the beginning of another. I don't carry it with me everywhere, but it sits on my writing desk at my cottage, where I can open it any time I want to find the words I need.

My favourite is Mary Oliver's "Wild Geese," and if you turn to the epigraph of this book, you will see why. Oliver's idea that you don't have to be good or repent, you just have to love what you love—even thinking about those words makes my heart tighten.

My near burnout was like the call of those geese, harsh and exciting. I needed it to rediscover my place in the family of things. Now I am once again able to do what I signed up for on that treadmill, the day MAiD became legal. I carry the burden of ending people's lives. It nearly made me fall apart. Now it's part of the glue that holds me together.

CHAPTER ELEVEN

Yolanda, Part Three

I gaped when I saw the email from Yolanda.

It was now March 2018. More than a year had passed since that afternoon at Patty's when she'd told me her story. I thought I'd seen her off into the arms of the team at University Health Network, a hospital system with a reputation for taking care of its own. I assumed she'd had her MAiD months ago.

Yet here was her note in my inbox, asking me if I remembered her. "Who ever could have forgotten you?" I said aloud.

As it turned out, she hadn't been ready the previous year. She was drawing down on her time, waiting until she was certain. Now she had a date, July 31. But she wanted to do it "right."

Over the next four months, Yolanda and I exchanged a number of emails—thirty-seven, to be exact. I sent thirty-five further emails to her various doctors. I saw Yolanda twice in hospital and twice more at Patty's. I know she matched my efforts stroke for stroke, even though she could only function four hours per day. Because true to her core, Yolanda left nothing to chance.

She was determined to donate her battered lungs to research, which meant that a transplant team had to be standing by to harvest them immediately after her death. But she didn't want to die in a hospital. Too cold. She was considering the Kensington Hospice, which was affiliated with UHN. But she was frustrated with her UHN caregivers. I suggested my home base, Women's College Hospital; she agreed to mull that over. Wherever it happened, she wanted all decisions made by mid-May, so she could spend June and July relaxing and saying goodbye to friends. "I just want to be present in the remainder of my life," she said.

She was distressed by how many of the logistics of her death were falling to her to organize. She was coordinating twenty-five people on different email chains: her palliative care doctors, her lung and renal specialists, me. The transplant team had agreed to take her lungs and kidneys for research, so she coordinated how her body would get to the hospital morgue. But who would receive her body there? Who would retrieve her organs, and how would her body get to a funeral home afterward? (She refused to burden her family with that last detail.) She offered to stop her oxygen so she would meet the requirement for admission to hospice:

imminent death. But what if doing that made her too ill to consent in the moment?

She was shouting for help as loudly as she could, but she wasn't being heard. And here I was again, the eternal squeaking wheel, rolling into a megalith hospital conglomerate that I wasn't a part of. Once again, I said something I had no business saying, promised something I didn't know if I could deliver: "I will make it work." But this time it was a promise to myself, too—if I couldn't make it work for Yolanda, I really had no business doing this. I *would* make it work.

I still had a glimmer of faith that the UHN team would pick up this ball and help me carry it over the line. So I called Dr. Madeline Li, the head of UHN's MAiD service. She was an ally, and savvy about navigating the many divisions and specialists that would be involved. She assured me that she knew of Yolanda's case and that things were in process; we assured each other that we had enough time to get this right. I phoned Yolanda, buoyant: she could have MAiD when she wanted at UHN; she just needed to sign a new formal request.

But Yolanda was still Yolanda—she wanted to investigate every option. Could I show her the MAiD set-up at Women's College? And could her parents and aunt come, too? I was flabbergasted: each time we had spoken, Yolanda mentioned that her mother, a devout Catholic, was so strongly against MAiD that she was terrified her daughter would burn in hell as a suicide.

"Really! She wants to come?" I asked. "And you're up for this?" My mind was racing.

"She's come round a bit since last June," Yolanda replied, "after I almost died with pneumonia."

Yolanda's mother still wouldn't attend her MAiD procedure, she added. And truth be told, Yolanda didn't want her to. She didn't think she'd be able to consent if her mother were there. But her mother did want to see where it might happen.

"My mother and other people in my family still cling to the hope for a miracle," Yolanda said. "I've almost convinced them that the miracle has happened: I've survived thirty years with this disease."

As it turned out, both mom and aunt had fond memories of the old Women's College. They marvelled at the renovation, the towering atrium, the stores. "Maybe we should shop," they joked, as we wheeled Yolanda by the jewellery store, Vivah. I told them that Avivah had been a patient of mine. An exquisite craftsperson, she sourced all her fresh water pearls, silver, and semi-precious stones from Asia, travelling there often. She had also been on the list for an organ transplant at UHN. I stopped short of noting that she was Yolanda's age when she died.

I was proud of the two MAiD rooms I'd secured, tucked away in the ambulatory urgent care unit—until I saw the flat look in Yolanda's eyes. "Can you describe exactly what happens?" she asked. Did she really want me to detail how I put in the IV lines, how I administer the drugs one by one? In front of her mother? Yes, she did. Now her face went brittle, her eyes dark.

That visit firmed her resolve: Yolanda wanted to die in a place she found peaceful. A hospital would not cut it. Patty offered her home, and Yolanda accepted.

I offered to take over the logistics of her organ donation. First call: Madeline Li again. "Who do I need to talk to at UHN?" The answer: R.J. Edralin, the nurse practitioner who was the MAiD coordinator. He's a busy man, travelling among four hospitals and the Kensington Hospice, trying to be present at every provision in all the locations, starting the IVs if needed, retrieving the drugs, coordinating the services, running the debriefs. In other words, my kind of guy.

Second call: Edralin, now and ever after R.J. He promised to make the retrieval of Yolanda's organs his priority— which meant booking the surgical team at Toronto General, ensuring that someone was on site to receive her body, and providing direction to pathology. The transport time from Patty's home to Toronto General would be about fifteen minutes, the same as if Yolanda's body were coming from the hospice. It should all work out, right? Right?

A new email from Yolanda arrived. She was coming down with a respiratory infection. Would that affect her eligibility to donate her lungs? Given that her last chest infection had nearly killed her, I alerted R.J. to prepare a plan B if Yolanda were admitted to Toronto General before she died. That might make the transplant logistics easier, but it would also cut me out of the process.

A week later, R.J. phoned back. With "creative shepherding," he said, he had sorted out a date that worked for all the necessary teams. Dr. Juvet, the head of the research team, wrote to assure me that a lung infection would not preclude donation of lung tissue. Yolanda had looped in her friend James, one of her powers of attorney for care. Though he lived in Vancouver, he promised to negotiate the minutiae of transfers and consents. Yolanda had to sign her own consent documents for autopsy and organ donation (that must have been tough). And I needed to know what time she wanted me to arrive on the day, and how many people might attend.

When I got her on the phone, however, I was surprised by the depth of unhappiness in Yolanda's thin, husky voice. She was finding the process "quite drawn out and much more complicated than a person who is exhausted needs it to be." No one at UHN had ever sat her down for a proper conversation about her end-of-life goals, she said.

"Not once in the six months that I have been telling people what my intent was," she said. "Westernized culture focuses on getting treatments—'It's available, try it!' We assume that more life is always the goal. But in my case, that hasn't been the goal for a long time. I don't want to keep living this way. The last two days it's been so nice out, but I haven't left the house. I don't have the stamina to fill my own oxygen tank and put it in my walker. My life is a regimen of pills and exercises. What's left for me is sitting in a home, fading away, and I'm going to skip that part.

"So now what I want is to relax and see the people I love, try to go to the beach, and be as free from a schedule as I can be. I want to be as chilled out as possible until it happens," she said. Instead, she was spending most of her time organizing her death.

She was dealing with another difficult task, too: she was managing her friends' grief. "Telling people that you're going to do MAiD creates a whole different set of burdens than passing away suddenly would," Yolanda said. People she loved, but who were not her nearest and dearest, were flying in from around the globe to spend time with her—and they wanted her to schedule their visits. They wanted to bring their small children, whom Yolanda didn't even know. They wanted hotel suggestions and restaurant recommendations. Some arrived without warning. Others would text her, and if she didn't respond quickly, they'd text back, "What's wrong?"

"What's wrong?" Yolanda repeated, exasperated. "I can't breathe!"

It made her kind of angry, frankly—their reactions were about themselves, not her. "They want to share their grief about me with me, constantly," she said. "I'm touched that I have so many friends who love me, but I don't want to spend my last weeks crying. I mean, I am sad; that's normal. But I don't want to spend my final days thinking only about my death. Believe me, I think about it enough. Every day I wake up thinking, I'm one day closer to it. Later today I'll probably stop at Mount Pleasant cemetery to see the niche my urn will be in.

"Every day, I make this choice," she continued. "It's not a choice I made once. Every day I think about it, and I always come to the same conclusion. I'm already dying. I'm not doing anything that isn't going to happen. I've had enough of trying my best."

I asked her what she did want from people, what people could do for her. I told her it would be useful for me to know this, so I could pass it on to other MAiD families. She rhymed off a ready list.

They can tell her how much they love her. That seems obvious, she said, but often it's assumed and not expressed. They can share stories about the impact they've had on each other. They can ask, "What do you need?" And if she's too tired to think of what she needs, they can offer ideas: I'll make you a meal, you eat it when you can. I'll mow your lawn. I'll clean your bathroom. If they invite her to dinner, they should make the arrangements. "Think of what a person likes," she summed up, "and do that." What she didn't need was to hear how excruciating it was for others to see her in this state.

Yolanda loved food of all kinds—whatever the opposite of food neophobic might be, that was her—so she created a food bucket list. It gave her friends something fun they could do for her. One friend brought her famous Asian dumplings; another treated her to a meal in her favourite restaurant. On our last visit—she'd invited me for four p.m. because she was having dinner guests at five—I offered to make a beet hummus we'd both read about in the *New York Times*. That made her happy, which made me happy.

By then, the extended visits and FaceTime goodbyes were winding down, and Yolanda was concentrating on what her last days should feel like. She wanted to see only her closest family and friends. She was "guested out" and finished with scheduling. "If I wake up on my second-last day on Earth and want to wander around a farmers' market, that's what I'll do," she said. "If I want to watch TV, I'll do that." Some friends thought she was "jumping the gun" because she didn't look especially frail; she was finished trying to convince them. "Death comes in all shapes and sizes," she said. Some of her mother's friends were still saying, "She won't go through with it." She was finished arguing.

She was even finished worrying about her organ donation. If July 31 wasn't going to work for the transplant team, she would forgo that request. She was prioritizing her needs now.

Happily, at the beginning of July, R.J. came through—all the players were in place for the 31st. He and I organized a meeting in a UHN conference room so everyone could go over the plan face to face. I arrived at the appointed time to find . . . no one. Only R.J. and me. I was stunned. He was apologetic. He'd prepared a PowerPoint presentation, and I sat through it in silence. He handed me a copy of the run sheet, which outlined estimated times of actions, relevant personnel, contact numbers. He'd even arranged for the transplant team to cover the cost of transporting Yolanda's body to the funeral home. I was impressed and told him so. But I was also seething. This massive institution, with all its resources, could not get it together to turn up, look at each other, and organize the last act of caring for this one tiny woman.

Then Yolanda had a final surprise for me: she wanted to talk to a spiritual counsellor. Could I help her find one? I knew Yolanda was a lapsed Catholic. I knew she had a psychiatrist, as well as a long-time social worker, Kristen, from when she lived in Boston. (In fact, part of the reason Yolanda had chosen July 31 for MAiD was so Kristen could attend.) But I had neglected to inquire about her spirituality. Though the hospital offered a questionnaire that she could submit, I wasn't able to find anyone suitable. I felt that I had let her down, and it cut deeply. I know these conversations matter. They need time to surface, time for reflection, for silent listening, compassion. Now there was no time left.

In our last conversation before her provision day, I asked Yolanda if she believed in an afterlife. Her answer, coming from a scientist, surprised me. "I don't know," she replied. "It would be arrogant to say a hard no. What we know is that we're always learning things." She had felt the presence of her grandfather on the night he died. She once sensed her late grandmother standing at the foot of her bed.

"I wish I could believe," she said. "I can understand why people are religious, or why they turn religious near the end. If it helps my parents to believe I'm going to heaven, what's the harm? I do believe that our bodies are energy, and whatever the next state will be, it's going to be peaceful. I'll be at peace, whether I know it or not."

She was certain of this: having MAiD as an option had given her a lot of comfort. She was grateful she wouldn't have to suffer. "If there is a God," she said, "I believe they'd be merciful. I believe they'd understand my choice."

On the morning of Yolanda's procedure, as the clock ticked past ten thirty while I waited for my nurse, Yuri, to arrive, I opened my backpack and took out a large rectangular box, the kit that contains the MAiD drugs and syringes. Deliberately, I turned my back to the room, my body shielding my actions, and set the box on the dining room table. I slit open the tape and began laying out the contents on a baking sheet.

Even though I wanted to hurry things along, I forced myself to slow down, be methodical. Every time I unwrapped a plastic package, I checked it off my list. Five large syringes for the MAiD drugs, check. Four smaller syringes for normal saline (to help push the drugs through the lines), check. I filled each syringe in turn (check, check, check). I noted the time, Yolanda's name, and ID number. I wrote down the names of a few of the many attendees, along with their phone numbers (the coroner would ask for this later). I moved with a practised rhythm, my concentration narrowed to a pinpoint. I checked my last mark and stood upright. I'd been crying earlier, when everyone was singing, but I wasn't just then.

Yuri sprinted through the door at about ten forty. (Bless him forever.) Looking out the front window, I could see that the hearse and attendants had arrived, too. They patiently waited outside on the porch, but it was a little ghoulish, another reminder that we were behind schedule to get Yolanda's body to the surgical team at UHN. I worried it would upset the witnesses.

I moved to Yolanda and whispered in her ear. "Okay, everyone into the kitchen," she called out. She turned to one friend who had told her he couldn't bear to watch the procedure itself. "Time for you to go upstairs," she said. She hugged him. She hugged everyone. Then she settled in a velvet armchair in a corner of the living room with her feet up on an ottoman, looking out the front window onto the street and the summer trees. "Here's my last quote," she said. "I'm surrounded by love and peace, and I've never felt more sure of my decision."

Yuri tried to find a vein for her IV, then tried again. (Could we not do one thing right by this woman?) "Can you use my port?" she asked calmly—meaning the permanent medicine tube that ran into her chest near her collarbone, a testament to her medication-filled years. Embarrassed to have missed that, we attached the line to the port and tucked the tubing behind Yolanda's back—again, so no one would have to see what was happening.

I perched on a low table at Yolanda's side. "I'm now going to ask for your consent," I said. I listed the facts: "You've been diagnosed with a rare lung disease. It's in an advanced stage. You've been told your alternatives. None are acceptable to you. You are suffering as a result of your condition. You are requesting assistance to die." I listed the drugs I was about to use—not every doctor does that, but I wanted Yolanda to know we were going to do this right. Finally I said, "You know this will result in your death. I will then call the coroner. Do you want me to proceed?"

Throughout, Yolanda regarded me steadily, her eyes brilliant, sparkling with intensity. Her voice, when she consented, was shaky but clear. To be thorough—thorough to the end—she also wrote out her consent.

Her friends came back into the room and arrayed themselves around her, some kneeling by her side, some standing. Everyone was crying and smiling, radiating love. Someone rubbed her feet. "I couldn't have asked for a better send-off," Yolanda said, looking each person in the eye. "Let's put on the final playlist."

Simple Minds' "Don't You (Forget About Me)" came on, followed by Coldplay's "Fix You," and other songs about exhaustion and farewell. Yolanda sang every word.

What she didn't see were the subtle looks that Yuri and I were exchanging, standing behind her. I had started with one syringe (10 cc's) of midazolam, the sedative. With each syringe, I would quietly note the time—midazolam, 11:04 a.m.—and Yuri would write it down. Midazolam is usually fast-acting. Administered through a port, it works even faster.

But Yolanda remained awake. At some point she closed her eyes, but she kept singing. Where she got that power, I don't know. Maybe it was because she'd been so practised in husbanding her energy. Maybe it was just her ferocious spirit. I flushed the tube with more saline. Yolanda kept singing.

I whispered to Yuri for the lidocaine. As I mentioned earlier, the anaesthetic numbs the vein walls so they're not irritated by the propofol, which burns going in. I didn't want her body to jerk, even if she was asleep.

Yuri volunteered to open the spare box of meds I'd brought to get more midazolam. (I always bring extra.)

"Let's wait a bit longer," I whispered back. I flushed in more saline. Discreetly, I moved my hands to the sides of Yolanda's neck. It was a comforting position, but it had a purpose, too: I was monitoring her pulse. Somewhere in the middle of "Route 66," Yolanda finally fell asleep. It seemed perfect that her last words were "Take that trip."

At 11:09 a.m., I administered the propofol, 1,000 mgs. (That's the really thick drug I mentioned in Joe's chapter.) Propofol induces a deep coma. For many patients, it's the fatal dose. Because of the density of the drug, I had to alternate syringes of propofol with syringes of saline. I'd learned to lean on the syringes as discreetly as I could, but it took about two minutes just to push it all in. After about five minutes, Yolanda's breathing was no longer visible.

But that wasn't the end. I could still feel her heart beating. At 11:14 a.m., I administered the final medication, rocuronium, the one that paralyzes the lungs. (I always use all the drugs, even if a patient is already gone.) Yuri and I continued our watch of Yolanda's pulse in her carotid artery. She'd been using so many muscles to breathe for so many years, her vessels were in bold relief.

I was worried the others could see Yolanda's pulse, too. But they weren't watching the procedure. They were crying and singing, looking into Yolanda's face, or down at the ground, or up at the ceiling. They were holding on to each other, and to her, touching whatever part of her was nearest, her knee, her ankle.

Yolanda was strong, I knew that. But she was even stronger than I'd estimated. I had put her in a deep coma. She would not be rousing. All I could do now was wait.

I've done scores of MAiD procedures. I know how to keep myself in check emotionally. I suspend what's in my head and concentrate on doing my job kindly and efficiently. My feelings aren't part of it; I keep them out of the way. But now I was crying again. I'd spent more time with Yolanda than with most MAiD patients. I felt moved by her family, the way they'd made this day into a ceremony, with music and dancing and tenderness. I knew that by providing MAiD I was doing what Yolanda wanted, but I also recognize its power. I don't think of this job as ending a life; I think of it as honouring it.

But standing there, my hands on Yolanda's delicate shoulders, I also felt guilt. I ran down the long list of how we'd failed her. All those emails that should have been unnecessary, the delays, even today's embarrassing flubs. (How did I not remember that she had a medicine port?)

I didn't know it then, but the missteps would continue after she died. I didn't know that Yolanda had told her aunt, in no uncertain terms, that she did not want to exit the house in a body bag. When the funeral home attendants came in with one on their gurney and began to zip it around her body, her distraught aunt came to me. "I'm sorry," I had to tell her. "I don't see how we can take her outside exposed."

I didn't know that Yolanda's uncle would phone me late that afternoon to say the funeral home still hadn't confirmed they had her body. I didn't know that I would end up calling the funeral home ready to fully rant, only to find out that when they'd arrived at the hospital morgue, no one was there to release her body. By then it was well after four p.m., and the staff at both locations were leaving for the day. I knew Yolanda's family needed her to be at the funeral home, so they could begin their arrangements for the service there. "Call them again," I would say to the funeral home coordinator, through gritted teeth. (Luckily, she would hear my desperation and make it happen.)

But I didn't expect the sweet moments, either. Waiting for the coroner to call back, I had a lot of time to talk to family members. They told me Yolanda had spent her last night in her father's arms, peaceful, consoled. I had no idea that her father would volunteer to be the witness who spoke to the coroner. I never imagined that he would say, "I struggled with Yolanda's decision. But now that I've seen it, I think if the time came, I would want MAiD for myself." That would nearly break me.

I wouldn't understand until later that Yolanda represented the best of my hopes for MAiD—that for the right person, it's an essential component of care—and she also represented the worst of my frustrations with MAiD's short-comings. We're doing a good thing. We have to do it better.

In the end, she led the way through her death, not me. Knowing her, I should have expected that.

When Yolanda's pulse finally stopped, I lifted my hands from her neck. Gently, gently, I removed her oxygen tube. I held a stethoscope to her chest. I looked at my watch. "Time of death," I said softly, "11:23 a.m."

CHAPTER TWELVE

Lessons Learned

So what have I learned from providing MAiD—about medicine, about being human, about myself? When I began doing this five years ago, that wasn't the kind of question I typically asked myself. But the ground has shifted regarding what we doctors understand we are doing when we help someone to die, and how we practise that assistance. And how I personally feel about it. It's shifting still.

Lesson one: people want the option of assisted death. As of this writing, of the 195 countries on Earth, nearly thirty jurisdictions in more than a dozen countries allow for it. In Canada, it is embedded in the Charter of Rights and Freedoms that ensures citizens their right of autonomy of body and person. And Canadians are exercising that right. By December 2020, less than four years after provisions became legal, over 21,000 Canadians had opted to die via MAiD—roughly 2.5 percent of all deaths in the country. And the numbers will surely continue to rise; in jurisdictions with longer histories of MAiD (for instance, the Benelux countries), assisted death ranges around 4 to 5 percent.

People also want MAiD to be easier to access, with fewer roadblocks. In March 2021, the Canadian Parliament complied by passing Bill C-7, which expands the eligibility criteria for MAiD.

I've talked a lot in this book about the RFND clause—natural death being reasonably foreseeable. I told you how we physicians vigorously debated, in our online CAMAP forums and in our own consciences, what *reasonably* and *foreseeable* meant and how we interpreted and applied that legislation. Diseases such as cancer, with defined clinical stages and a perceptible trajectory to death, gave us parameters that were crisp and clear for those cases. But many other diseases and illnesses are too murky for us to predict the progression to death.

By the end of our first annual CAMAP conference in Victoria in 2017, we agreed that clinical practice guidelines for RFND were essential, and we developed them. These guidelines not only give us comfort; they also allow us flexibility in how we reckon death is likely to occur in the not-too-remote future. In other words, if a patient's death is predictable, they don't have to be actively dying in order to be eligible for MAiD. We've worked successfully within this framework for five years.

We even used those principles to work within the guidelines for patients with cognitive decline, the murkiest condition of all. Alzheimer's, for example, is a fatal disease with a predictable trajectory to death within five to ten years. So using that guideline, without specifying exactly when death will occur, I was able to assess and find patients eligible for MAiD. I followed these people carefully, and when it appeared that capacity was about to be lost, I stepped in to advise them and their families that the time to set a date, to act on their wishes for a dignified exit, had arrived. They could withdraw their request—every patient has that right—but if they wanted to go ahead, I would let them know that their consent was now essential, before they lost the capacity to understand and reason through the consequences of their ask.

Since March 2021, under Bill C-7, that framework has widened. There now are two tracks to assisted death: track one is pretty much what we've been doing with a few updates. Patients' natural deaths still must be reasonably foreseeable. However, they are no longer required to wait ten days after requesting MAiD for a provision; they now need only one witness to their death, rather than two; and some patients no longer have to be able to give consent on the day itself.

That last one is a biggie: it ensures, by a written agreement between the patient and the provider, that a patient who's been approved for MAiD won't be denied it if they lose mental capacity before a provider can carry it out—for example, via a stroke, a sudden intensification of dementia, or escalating opioid dosage for pain management.

That agreement is called the waiver of final consent (WFC). It is *not* the same thing as an advance directive, or a living will. Instead, it's a written agreement between an eligible patient and provider; it specifies an agreed-upon provision date. On that date, a patient doesn't have to remember what they had for breakfast. They don't even have to remember my name. However, if they show any refusal in words, gestures, or sounds to the administration of the drugs, I do not proceed. If they retain capacity and are able to sign another waiver, the date can be moved forward. It's more work for doctors, and it may add confusion to a patient's already shaky understanding. But for me— and for so many families out there—it's worth it.

Gordon is a good example of how the updates will allow track one patients to breathe a bit easier. He was ninety when I met him, living in a small condo in the heart of Toronto. It was March 2020, days before the first COVID-19 lockdown. None of us wore masks. His twin daughters, who lived a few blocks away, hovered.

Gordon, though slight, was a spry, energized, amiable character. He bubbled with stories about his years as a cub reporter on the Prairies, his thirty-odd avocations, including insurance salesman and art broker—in short, his full, fantastic life. "It has been a challenge and an adventure," he said.

A minute later, he said it again, because his short-term memory was shot. He was caught in an endless repetition of story, rewind, story. But he was clear about one thing: he wanted an assisted death when the time came. "I have a fantastic life," he boomed. "My girls are looking after me very well. But when the time comes . . ."

How soon, though, would that time have to be? He'd already had a serious fall on the street (miraculously, it didn't land him in hospital, despite his osteoporosis). His decreased appetite and weight loss had made him skeletal. His daughters had taken away his car keys and his liquor. Ever cheerful, he accepted ice cream instead. His daughters and I fretted that if Gordon waited too much longer, he would no longer have the capacity to consent. I knew it would be a close call. Then as I was leaving, he rushed up. "Is it today?" he asked. Not exactly reassuring.

As we sank under the weight of COVID and the year wore on, I checked in regularly with Gordon via Zoom. He stayed steady, reassuring me that his life was good and he was happy and well cared for. It wasn't time yet.

Then one morning, he went to the concierge in his building. Something was wrong with his phone. He couldn't get it to work.

There was nothing wrong with the phone. He just couldn't remember how to work it. The daughters called, and we arranged another assessment. It was time. "I am ready," he said.

On the day of Gordon's provision, I arrived at his condo in full personal protective equipment (PPE). "I know you, don't I?" he asked.

"Yes, Gordon, sorry about the regalia," I replied. "But can you tell me what I am here to do for you today?"

"You're here to put me down," he said. And then he was off again about his good life. Relief washed over me.

His daughters were weeping—had been for days. They climbed onto his bed and took his hands as he stretched out, spiffy in a neat shirt and cords. They kissed him and wiped their eyes and told him they would love him forever. He had a lot to say to them, too. They were his treasures for every minute of his life. He was leaving them a bit of money, not much but something. He wanted them to know how much it mattered that he could help them out.

"Gordon?" I asked during a promising pause. "Do you want me to go ahead with the needle now?"

"Yes, go ahead," he said. As I began, he turned back to his daughters and talked some more. Until quiet filled the room.

It was a good death.

While it isn't always easy or comfortable to follow patients who are losing their mental faculties, Gordon is a shining example of how it can be done. We imagine mental decline as a gradual creep; we imagine we'll be able to spot the moment it's about to turn. But waiting for MAiD is more an act of faith. Anything can happen at any moment to derail one's intentions—a life-threatening stroke, an incapacitating fall. Gordon and his daughters lived with the risk of missing his window of capacity. He was lucky. He enjoyed one extra year and still had his good death. With the WFC, patients like Gordon and their families don't have to worry so much about missing their window. They don't have to rely on luck. Sheila and Lisa, I'm thinking of you.

I want to be clear here: I prefer to monitor patients, to walk the distance until it is time, and then to look them in the eyes and know that they know what I am there to do. But for patients whose condition may suddenly change, the WFC is a godsend, to patient and doctor both. It's often referred to as Audrey's amendment to honour Audrey Parker, who received MAiD in 2018, sooner than she wished because she feared that her breast cancer, which had spread to her brain, might prevent her from consenting on a later date. None of us wants that.

So, that is track one. Track two is even bigger news.

Track two patients are those whose natural death has not yet become reasonably foreseeable but who still meet the eligibility criteria outlined for all patients: they have a serious illness, disease, or disability; they are in an advanced state of irreversible decline in capability; that illness, disease, disability, or decline in capability is causing them enduring, intolerable, and irremediable suffering; and they have given consent after having been informed about all available means of help or assistance—including palliative care. But their natural death need no longer be reasonably foreseeable.

Track two requires patients to wait ninety days from request to provision, during which time all available means of social, physical, disability, and mental health services must be laid out and seriously considered, and the assessors must consult experts in the patient's condition if they themselves do not have expertise in it. Once those requirements have been fulfilled, the clinician is legally permitted to provide MAiD. But a new crop of issues will invariably arise.

For example, should plain old age open the door to considering a request for an assisted death if an elder believes that the irreversible decline in their capability is causing them irremediable suffering? And if so, is it sufficient reason to request or receive an assisted death? With track two, the answer possibly can be yes. Given Canada's aging population, more of our elders—isolated, lonely, dependent for the barest of needs, warehoused in long-term care homes—may see MAiD as a relief from that version of suffering. We saw hints of it during COVID: devastating declines in cognition; a loss of connection and purpose; the sense that life had no meaning. We should get ready.

And there's more. As of March 2023, track two should have included MD-SUMC—mental disorder as the sole underlying medical cause for a MAiD request. As of this writing, controversy and debate are raging around MD-SUMC, and not only because if it becomes law, Canada will have the most liberal assisted death legislation in the world. (Already we are leagues ahead of most jurisdictions, even without the mental illness clause.) Determining eligibility with MD-SUMC will be difficult and taxing. Our CAMAP forums will once again be on fire with questions and doubts. Already the way ahead is looking very different from the path behind. The sunset clause that was to have permitted MD-SUMC has been advanced to March 2024.

As everyone does, I wrestle with issues about the value, meaning, and purpose of a life. But my work requires me to make those determinations concrete about others' lives. So I dig into many sources for my affirmation and solace.

In his 2015 book *Homo Deus: A Brief History of Tomorrow*, Yuval Harari considers how humanity might conquer death itself. It starts, he says, with replacing body parts, and ends with replacing minds with artificial intelligence. The cost is that we lose the meaning of the value of life.

In his argument, liberal humanism has replaced religion, socialism, and capitalism as the underpinnings of belief. We no longer must live a good life to be rewarded in an afterlife. We no longer even expect there is one. Nor do national identity and collective responsibility hold sway over individualism. Rather, the value of your life rests on your shoulders. If you are in an existential crisis about why you exist, or what the meaning of life is, or when and how it should end, you may find yourself in the unhappy position of being your own sole arbiter. That's a lot to bear alone. Not even Yolanda, the consummate analyst, wanted to tackle that.

But humanism is also the core of the argument upon which Bill C-7 rests: we all die. Old age is a terminal state for everyone who makes it that far. And suffering can be intolerable long before it's fatal. Very few people increase their capabilities as they age or grow sicker. So if you are suffering grievously, and if the value of your life is solely up to you, you may request an assisted death, and we doctors may feel obligated to help you.

Lesson two: our community can do a lot better. The COVID-19 pandemic exposed, to our shame, how we as a country and a society demean our elderly. It showed us in grim detail how lean our care has become after decades of diverted funding, understaffing, and dependence on families (especially women) to keep the system going. Ninety percent of the deaths in the early months of the first wave were in this age group. *Ninety percent.*

There was one dim light through those first catastrophic months, as viral spread decimated seniors in long-term care homes: publicly funded homes did better than those that were privately run. Marginally! But enough to show us that more thoughtful staffing models, with more measured and accountable patient care hours, had better protected frail elders.

So will Canada's provinces heed that lesson going forward? Legislative action has been tabled in Ontario: to raise the bar of direct patient care to three hours per day and to reduce congestion and give each patient more room. But that is the bottom rung of what is needed if we want to care for our elders with actions and not sentiment. So many people need round-the-clock care. So many will never get it.

In my years of doing MAiD, one of the most harrowing things I've learned is just how many people are alone out there. How many people outlive their friends, their families. How lingering illness eventually wears down and chases away even the most well-intentioned friends.

How did we allow caring for our elders and our ill to become a rarity, rather than a basic tenet of society? What does that mean for the future of us as human beings? If we continue down this road, warehousing our seniors and our sickly in institutions where they are left alone, encouraged to use wheelchairs early to prevent falls, counting down the hours until death, we are setting up the perfect storm for what some predict will amount to an "easier out." I believe in MAiD, but I fear and abhor this kind of future for our seniors.

Don't get me wrong: I see excellent care being provided to frail elders and the chronically ill in hospitals and long-term care facilities. I see dedicated volunteer workers and paid staff who care for family or strangers with complicated bodily needs and often hollowed-out minds. They should be acknowledged for their value and purpose. Like Tom's nurse, they are the quiet champions—maybe not so quiet now, in the COVID era—and defenders of the vulnerable.

But I also see how care needs escalate with patients over time. I see in family members and caregivers how fear and fatigue march in step with sadness, grief, and loneliness. Not only can dying itself be a messy thing, but it is also challenging for families who bear the brunt of caring for an ailing loved one without a break, who are ever alert for a sudden calamity, and who are at the greatest risk of burning out themselves.

I'm eighty, and the perception of old age as a terminal state is a particular sensitivity of mine. Oh, I'm aware of my small deficits, my willingness to do a little less, my gratitude for a little more help. But I balk when anyone assumes that means my capabilities are faltering.

Perhaps that's why I declined, pre-track two, the MAiD request of a woman I'll call Enid. She was ninety-four. She lived independently in a retirement residence. She drove herself to my office. My nurse was agog at her youthful appearance. "She looks like a sixty-year-old Marilyn Monroe," she pronounced loudly as she brought her down the hall to me. (She never brought patients down the hall.) I gave Enid an examination, which grew more thorough the longer I could find nothing wrong with her. No comorbidities. Clean bloodwork. She was in every sense hale, capable, cognitively sharp—and extremely put out with me. Because she wanted MAiD. She'd lived her life well, but it was done. She was lonely, despite an extended family. She wanted release.

Enid met Harari's definition of the individual as the prime determinate of the value of her life. And the death of any ninety-four-year-old is foreseeable. But she didn't meet *my* criteria for approving MAiD. My roots are sunk in obligation and duty of care. They bend to societal rather than humanist precepts. Enid was at an advanced age, but she did not have an advanced illness. My moral centre, which held that her life still had value and purpose, did not find her reason to die ("I'm tired") reason enough. I told Enid I'd keep her file open and keep in touch.

Later, I regaled a colleague with the story of Enid and her glowing health. "You should have sent her to me," the doctor said sternly. "You owed that to her. I would have approved her."

I was gobsmacked. "On what basis?" I asked.

"On the basis of her life lived," she replied. We agreed to disagree.

For the first few years of my MAiD practice, I would spend sleepless nights wrangling with my conscience about issues like this. Had we done enough for the patient? What if there were more supports? I told myself that if I was losing sleep, I was probably asking the right questions. I was probably doing my patient justice.

Now I wonder if my experience, coupled with the new legislation, is leading me to a fresh rash of sleepless nights. Have I reached a place where my moral distress at our collective failures is interfering with a patient's right to ask for death?

These track two cases are difficult to parse. The easy thing for me would be to pass them on to another assessor, who likely will give the patient what they want. Of course, then I slam up against another issue: the shallowness of the pool of assessors and providers. I know most of them, and they know me. We desperately need more doctors to join us. Because things are going to get messy.

Part of my discomfort with track two stems from lesson three: just because we can do MAiD, that doesn't mean we should. So many times, a patient who's asked me to assess them will say they have one more treatment to try, or child to see brought into this world, or Christmas to experience. At that point, I nod: they don't need me yet. But they do need people to be with them. And at the end, what they may need is a vigil, not MAiD.

I'm still troubled by one of my provisions, a woman I'll call Sarah. Her palliative doctor had gone to visit her at home, and alarmed by Sarah's precipitous decline, called me. "Can you do this provision in the next day or two?" I scrambled, but when I got there, Sarah was barely rousable. Her three grown sons had assembled. I could see they were acutely distressed with how fast this was happening. I flew in, feeling like the angel of death, provided for her, phoned the coroner, and left.

Now, a few years on, I might do it differently. I might say to her sons, "Do you really want me to do this? Or do you simply need to be here with her, sit with her, and let her death happen?" I worry that I took away something that those men should have had: time to be still with their dying mum.

I also think about the patient I'll call Earl. He'd been in chronic pain for ten years and was steadily losing ground. But as a recovered addict, he was struggling against taking opioid pain meds. He lived alone in Sudbury in assisted housing, and for a few brief hours a week, paid workers came to help him cook, clean, and do laundry. The more I talked to him, the less convinced I was that he was ready for MAiD. I told him there was new thinking around the drug ketamine for pain management. What if I could get him into a ketamine trial? He agreed to wait.

A few months later he called, frustration tightening his voice. "No one has called me about this trial!" he said. He was sick of waiting. He wanted MAiD now. I told him I'd call in favours; I'd get him more services. But I'd already dangled his eligibility for MAiD like a carrot in front of his nose, and he was eligible to receive it. I can rant all I want about social injustice, about the lack of services in smaller cities and rural areas, about the inequities that leave so many people like Earl feeling as if they have no other choice. But it's his decision, and it's our duty to provide if he is eligible. In the end, he did have a ketamine trial; it was ineffective. He proceeded with his goal to have MAiD. We arranged for a transfer to hospital so that he was able to donate his organs, a fitting legacy that pleased him no end.

As of this writing, I have not yet done a track two provision. But I did sort of finesse one: during the long COVID shutdown, I moved a patient from track two to track one. I'll call her Judith. She was an artist and an events coordinator; she once led art tours in Europe and lived in a gorgeous apartment with a massive art collection. I first assessed her in November 2020 via Zoom. The longer we talked, the less certain she seemed about MAiD. But she kept saying things that alarmed me. She was selling her art collection. Her apartment was so expensive. The lease was coming up. Was she asking to die because she was running out of money? Her long-time physician certainly held that view.

In summer 2021, when things had opened up COVID-wise, I visited Judith in person. Her niece and grandnephew were there. They assured me the family had a fund that would cover her expenses. As I caught up on her medical history, Judith admitted something new: she'd been having drop attacks, fainting spells presumably caused by sudden bouts of cardiac arrhythmia. She'd wake up on the floor, unaware of how she'd gotten there. She had not told her doctor.

"This warrants an investigation, Judith," I told her. "There are medications, treatment." She shook her head. She wanted no more tests, no more doctors. I took her blood pressure: 185 systolic. That put her at risk for stroke and for a lot of other hazards. Combined, those things were enough for me to shift her to track one.

There was a hitch, though: the assessor who'd seen her before me had deemed her track two. She'd have to wait ninety days for MAiD. But her lease was up September 1. She didn't want to wait.

So I did what I never do. I asked for a reassessment from a previous assessor. Usually, I viewed that as squandering of already-tight resources—but here it was necessary. We had new information. The assessor examined Judith and agreed she was track one. No waiting period. I provided for her on August 31.

Do you see what I mean about messy?

One thing you can count on if you provide MAiD: you will see the best and the worst of human nature. You will see families with unfinished business, with resentments both simmering and boiling over. You will see immediately which child is loved the most and which feels the most overlooked. Despite all that, MAiD can bring families together in a way that waiting out an unpredictable natural death cannot. That's lesson four: MAiD can be beautiful.

When my patients announce their intention to seek MAiD, their loved ones are, of course, pained. But rarely do they question the decision. Mainly, I see trust—if you've requested help to die, you must have thought it through. You must really need it. So there is respect and solidarity. People step up. Brothers, sisters, children do what's necessary. They make schedules, drive each other places, feed each other. They carve out time to visit, reminisce. MAiD gives families the opportunity to settle the kind of accounts I mentioned above, to say what needs saying, and to do it now. It's often awkward. But at the very least the door is open for one last chance to redress wrongs and make amends. I've seen the truth of this with Joe and with Tom. Family rifts are put to rest in the moment when what matters most moves to the fore, when a loving memory can replace a past hurt.

On provision day, generations gather. Babies are presented in arms for the last kiss. I've heard sermons delivered to crowds of relatives. I've attended a true Irish wake, sitting beside its subject. I've seen parents enfold their dying grown children and not weep until they are gone, to spare them the wailing. Such fortitude, such strength.

Lesson five is a corollary to four, only from the medics' perspective: we in the medical profession all need each other, too, whether we agree with MAiD or not. In my first seven years of provisions, I had my share of clashes with those who believe that if we can get quality palliative care sorted out, no one will need a MAiD provider. And yet I've seen so much good in a team approach.

After Joe's provision, my first, I had a long talk with the nurse who aided me. She spoke about her work in the intensive care unit—how much she valued her patients' lives, giving them her all in dedicated, unflinching care, but also how conflicted she sometimes felt when maintaining those lives with no hope for recovery.

I've worked hand in glove with the palliative teams at institutions that don't allow MAiD, such as Catholic hospitals and faith-influenced nursing homes. These teams, too, respect their patients' wishes. Acting within their own consciences, they go out of their way to arrange the transfer of a patient out of their institutions, IV lines intact, so that I am able to provide, either promptly on their arrival home or at my hospital, as we did with Thor.

Remember that I spent a year and a half in palliative care settings. As an assessor, that taught me to ensure, before I approve anyone, that a meaningful attempt to ease their suffering has been offered, expedited, or obtained. That is crucially important to me, even where the trajectory to death is obvious. Thanks to my self-administered educational program, I know when pain-relieving measures are inadequate. I recognize caregiver burnout. I feel when adequate support is lacking. I know how to—and still do—roll up my sleeves and get to work nursing desperately ill patients. I know when to put down my bag of drugs and sit with a dying patient and keep vigil as life ebbs away. This is the knowledge that sticks, that surfaces again and again when I take that rare moment to reflect. It also comes slamming back when I feel frustration or doubt about what to do next or where to turn for help.

Sometimes I know there is no answer. The turmoil I feel over a particular patient's decision is often my own. Did I do enough? Did we do enough? That's about my moral burden, my doubt. I've learned not to load that on my patients. I have to work that out on my own.

Thankfully, I know that I'm not the only MAiD provider who wrestles with these questions. I think back often to the early years of the CAMAP forums, where as a group, we focused on practicalities. Our conversations have evolved, and our forums are now flooded with discussions about moral conundrums. I don't think I'll be the last doctor who "just gets on with things," leaving her doubts unspoken, until they bring her to a precipice. But I'm comforted to know that the support, validation, and goodwill of the forum will allow MAiD providers to rededicate ourselves to the spirit and value of the work, the same way we bolstered each other with facts in the early years.

Near the beginning of the COVID lockdown in 2020, I drove the two hours from my cottage into Toronto, picked up the drugs, and went to end the life of my patient of forty years, Gayle. Her ovarian cancer was already widespread when we detected it, fatigue and bloat the ubiquitous symptoms. True to her bedrock, give-it-to-me-straight nature, she rejected aggressive surgery and chemo, instead opting for a second-line drug that would ease her pain and ensure the quality of life she sought. It bought her an extra eight months.

But the time had come, and there I was in full PPE, backpack in hand, at her home. Her husband and two adult daughters (one pregnant) were quietly distraught. A long-time labour organizer, Gayle had met life with teeth bared and a raucous booming laugh. One of her daughters, who'd grown up chronically and suicidally depressed, had been bullied and ostracized. Gayle had been a fierce advocate for her, storming the walls of bureaucracy, first to ensure her child's graduation from university, then to secure supported housing for her. She was equally determined to end her life her way. That day, shrunken except for her huge belly, her smile wan, with her girls and husband weeping nearby, she looked up at me and said simply, "Now."

Afterward, I didn't spend much time with Gayle's family. I blamed COVID—it robbed us of the chance to hug and to linger together. But the truth was I couldn't find words that would have felt adequate. I loved Gayle, too. I left quickly and sat in my car to report her death to the coroner. "She was my patient for almost forty years," I told the nurse practitioner.

"Oh, that must have been so hard for you," she replied.

And then I wept. It's the moments of tenderness, medic to medic, that can crack me open. Because we know what the other is feeling. The illness, pain, and death of our patients—it's hard for us, too.

I think often about the trauma that acute-care nurses and doctors have been experiencing, especially during COVID-19 surges. With chaos swirling around them, there is little time to feel, much less to talk about it. They are too busy rolling up their sleeves, working double and triple shifts. They dash between gurneys lined up in hallways as patients die in front of their eyes, even before they can attempt to relieve the patient's terror or suffering. Sometimes they find a patch of bare floor, lie down on it for a moment, and try to breathe their bodies into the solidity of the earth below. Sometimes they pass another worker, grab one of their hands, and squeeze, just for a second, exhausted beyond words, pushing ahead.

Emotions are an interference for a doctor; they can block necessary action. You get very good at burying them, layer after layer. You compress them into a shield. You teach yourself to feel less and less. In my early days of MAiD, if a feeling crept over me, I'd work harder. I'd make ten more calls; I'd pull in more services. I would combat my doubts with busyness, often passing the boundaries of reasonable effort. Anything to bury the emotional burden of the outcome: that I was the one who would end a life.

After the first CAMAP conference in 2017, I asked a psychiatrist for "some help." The ask wasn't clear or well framed. I didn't know how much trouble I was in then. She listened intently and suggested a book, a dense treatise on moral dilemmas by Lisa Tessman titled *When Doing the Right Thing Is Impossible*.

The paradox was too much for me—I'd begin to read it and immediately fall asleep, a perfect defence mechanism.

I do recall Tessman's example of the horrific situation that the doctors at Memorial Medical Center in New Orleans faced during Hurricane Katrina, when they realized they couldn't save everybody. (I'd think of it again in the haunting early days of COVID.) But back then, I couldn't see how it applied to me. It didn't offer solace or help me figure out what to do with my agitation. That would only dawn when Andrea Frolic equated my practising MAiD with high-risk medicine.

Now I understand why Gayle's death was so hard for me, and why the pileup of names and faces in the notebooks I keep of my MAiD provisions precipitated my crash. For me to work best, and for my work to be meaningful to me, I must feel a connection with the patients I serve. It is anathema to me to forget who they are, to not know their whole story, to not understand deeply what has propelled their request. I need to know who they touch in their lives, who loves them, whom they love. My comfort lies in being able to estimate how they value the life they've lived. In other words, I have to care about them.

Here's where the impossibility lies. Because at the same time, for me to be able to do this work, I have to silo off those feelings. I have to come to care about someone, and then I have to end their life. In the early days, I told myself that my moral distress was somehow reassuring. What didn't register was the cumulative burden, a wave that rose drop by drop. Until I nearly drowned in it, I didn't know how to pause and replenish.

So, lesson six: we can't only teach doctors how to do MAiD. We have to teach them how to survive doing it. Efficiency is good and necessary, as is perfecting the administration of the drugs. But if that is all we teach, I will not be the last person who burns out in this work. The solution is not to hive off MAiD providers into some elite subspecialty. The solution is to teach everyone to do it. And to give them permission to feel whatever they feel as they do it.

To feel the mess of it: the rawness and the relief, the effort of the work and the fear of failing (your patient, their family, your colleagues), the sadness and the surety, the taking of a life and the giving of peace.

CHAPTER THIRTEEN

A Good Death

A good death doesn't just happen.

For one thing, the timing has to be right. Every family asks me the same question: when exactly is that right time? I tell them I'm not a seer, much as I wish I were. I advise generalities and ask them to determine the specifics. A patient can't be too healthy or too far gone. They should feel some acceptance that the best is over and that what lies ahead is unwelcome.

For patients who are prepared to endure a long slow decline, I assure them that I will carry their file open for months, even years. For those with cancer, or end-stage heart disease, or failing memory, I watch them closely and repeatedly evaluate their current state. It requires reading between the lines of conversations that occur in hospital clinics: What messages have been communicated? Is futile hope being offered? Or is the slimness of the hope made clear, but the family hears only what they want? And now, with the added insurance of the waiver of final consent, I can ease a family's doubt about stretching the timeline too far, so they can rely on an exit for their loved one that ensures dignity and choice.

Hope clings tenaciously to us. Even for very ill patients, hope will override suffering. End-of-life conversations in the cardiac and nephrology clinics are notorious for being too little, too late. Even in the cancer clinics, when the "We've run out of options" conversation occurs, a family's fallback is often a variation of "The doctors said two to three months, and that was four months ago!" People want to cheat death, even by weeks. The question that I think is most important—How do you envision the last days of your life, and what would you want?—gets swept away by a litany of medical procedures and endless trips in and out of hospital.

As well, those who turn down further treatment often feel immediate dismissal, when what they need is a smooth transition to a palliative team. Palliation should not compete with active treatment in those clinics, but it is often read that way. After all, the notion of preparing to die while we are actively treating you runs counter to conventional wisdom. Yolanda, I'm thinking of you.

So yes, timing is critical. Once that has been set, though, the best death is often one that permits family, friends, and the patient to share a living wake. Knowing the date and time of the event obviates a lot of the shock and rue that can permeate funerals. There is time for gifts to children and mementos to grandchildren, visits from old friends and tender moments you could never summon or predict. And on the day of, MAiD allows people to say the things they want to say, while those who matter can still hear them. Meaningful memories are shared. Necessary thanks are given. Rifts are forgiven. Songs are sung, stories told. There's always laughter, a surprising amount, and it nourishes everyone there.

I look forward to hearing a patient's last words. I love how similar they turn out to be. Look after one another. Be good to each other. Remember me well, but don't worry about me. I had a good life. I am ready to go.

And sometimes a good death is not needing me at all. One morning, I arrived to do a provision for an elderly woman I'll call Edith. As I entered, her caregiver of twenty years exited. As a Catholic, she was not going to be in that room. It was just going to be Edith and me. But as I approached Edith, I saw that she wasn't conscious. I knew I wasn't going to administer the drugs; she couldn't give consent.

I sat down. I could feel her death coming. I am where I need to be, I thought. And there I stayed for an hour, watching her breathe. At some point I took out the nasal prongs delivering oxygen. She was at peace. Her breathing slowed. Then stopped. That was a good death, too.

Seven years in, I'm committed to doing this work, and absorbing all the changes that will come with advance requests and mental disorders as a sole underlying cause. Yet I know when a patient's death is also a good death for me. For me, the ultimate good MAiD death is a patient who has clarity of mind and knows that ending suffering is in their own hands. As of this writing, I'm not at the point where I feel certain I will be able to walk in on someone who cannot express consent and take their life. My use of the WFC so far has been very specific: it covers the predictable unforeseen events, such as a stroke or a metastatic progression that robs reason before I can provide the assisted death. I limit the timeline to two to three months at most. When we get to the appointed date, I insist on a review to determine if we can add more time and reset the date again. If there is no meaningful exchange between the patient and me at that time, I'm not sure I'd be able to take their life. I'm okay with being unsure. Like everything in this journey, the bridges we are building are crossed in the moment.

As well, I call a death *good* when I feel the patient's connections. When I feel they've had adequate family and community support, when they've been able to access sufficient disability support services, when their pain management has been optimal. The provisions that haunt me are the ones in which I sat in the home of the patient whose life I had just ended, waiting for the coroner's call, alone. Only me there to mourn them, or wish them on to a better place, or mark their star in the firmament. Unsure if their aloneness, rather than their illness or condition, was the real reason I was there.

I have profound respect for end-of-life caregivers. But in my first years of providing MAiD, I worried that my job—ending their patients' lives—invalidated their contribution in some unspoken way. My encounter with Tom's PSW changed the way I approach this work. It changed me. It made me reconsider what I was providing. What if I had been able to give Tom more connection to people, rather than just more pain meds? What if my first conversations had been with his support workers and not specialists?

These days, when I arrive to do an assessment or provision, I search the faces of my patient's caregivers. I am looking for affirmation, I am sure of that. I am seeking their participation in our goal to relieve this patient's suffering. And I am attesting that their caregiving hasn't been in vain.

For MAiD to continue working for me, I know that community services and resources must increase. Not everyone agrees with me. Some colleagues assure me that it's not my job to find these services for a patient, or even to say that someone must have them if they aren't available. With the advent of track two patient requests, assessors are tasked officially with reviewing the means that have been used to relieve suffering, including "counselling services, mental health and disability support services, community services, and palliative care." The law states that the patient "has been offered consultations with relevant professionals who provide those services or that care."

I'm all for that—but. The legislation also includes the phrase "where available," which does not mean that these things are available. Not even that they must be. "Those are social justice issues," my colleagues advise me. "Remote service disparities exist. Your obligation lies elsewhere."

But for me they go hand in hand. Advocacy and sourcing services are paramount and obligatory. So I nod my agreement when the Toronto-based cop who is the brother of my out-of-city patient says, "Forgive me, Doc, but I view the service base in northern Ontario as a backwater. I know the university hospitals on Avenue Road. I know the treatment clinics and the services that my brother could have here." I tell him that sourcing these services is my job, and we have been doing our due diligence together. It reassures him. It reassures me. My reward for reaching out for help for these patients is that—often to my surprise—it comes. People want to help, to try. That is good enough for me.

The legacy of isolation became painfully clear to me in 2020 and 2021 during the COVID-19 pandemic. Initially, MAiD requests decreased. Everyone went to ground, hunkered in, tried to stay well, stay alive. But after a few months, requests for provisions began to increase—first to the level in 2019, and then beyond. We've always anticipated that MAiD deaths will increase year by year until they reach a similar percentage to that in other jurisdictions, but this surge felt representative of something we already suspected. For our frail elders and those in nursing homes, isolation has devastating effects. What is the point of living longer if you're not able to hug your loved ones, to touch anyone, to sit with a fellow human and talk face to face? Elders deteriorated cognitively, physically. If anything, the pandemic reaffirmed that the values of living often lie in a simple connection to other human beings. When even that basic thread was severed, we saw patient requests magnify.

The rules say that every Ontarian must have equal access to palliative care—but they don't. The rules say that every Ontarian can access robust disability support—but they can't. The MAiD legislation, as written, says that all I'm obliged to do is make sure I have offered a patient what's available to them. If what they want is not available, the law says, it is not my concern. If a person requests MAiD solely because they can't get out of bed without help, and there is no one to assist, or a worker comes only two hours a day and that's not enough, well, that is our disgrace.

So I scramble. I send emails and make calls to reconnect a patient to someone, anyone in their circle. I reach for threads. I listen for clues. I will ask a patient and ask again, "What is your family doctor—or chronic pain specialist, or mental health clinic, or community resource centre—doing for you? What about that friend who did that smoke ceremony in your apartment that one time—can you reach out to her again?"

If the only reason I'm providing MAiD is that it's easier to die than it is to get decent, deserved help, then I risk being merely an expedient solution. I simply won't be that.

Even at my lowest, when I was sinking in the emotional mud and pulling back from MAiD, when someone called for me, I still stepped up. I always did. But I had to figure out what was eating me alive. So, to anyone considering this work: you have to really know yourself. After more than forty-five years on the job, I never imagined I could become as undone as I was during my modest breakdown. I think now that I was resisting what I knew to be true: I had to learn to accept that sometimes I was doing MAiD because the chain of care had failed. My loss; society's loss.

I know I will have to face that all over again, as the MAiD law evolves. Now that a person need not be dying to qualify for MAiD, assessors and providers will have to pick our way even more carefully through the moral minefield. The upcoming MD-SUMC clause—mental disorder as the sole underling reason to request MAiD—will be the toughest line we doctors walk. Human life is untidy. No one is the soul of perfection. Depression underlies or lingers, and drug use and addiction are often in the mix. But clinicians note that in studies of treatment-resistant depression, some 33 percent will improve on their own without further obvious interventions. How will I know if my patient is in the 66 percent that won't? How will these patients access newer therapies such as psychedelic psychotherapy and centres of healing? Who will pay? Who will do the work?

Moral distress has always been a cost to MAiD providers. It has become a repeated theme in our CAMAP forums and symposia over the years. Come March 2024, when the mental disorder clause in Bill C-7 comes into effect, it will fall to us—again—to tease out what the new legislation means for patients on the ground. I may think that a decision I make is "correct," but is it right? How can we know? It will fall to us to use, as the ethicist Kevin Reel calls it, "our last best judgment."

I first encountered Kevin at a (virtual) CAMAP symposium late in 2021. I was riveted by him and his story. Even on screen, he's open and warm. He shifts from chat to reflection, from narrative to morality, with fluid grace and a Yoda-like calm. He grew up in Canada and became an occupational therapist. While still a student, he helped initiate a home-based service for AIDS patients: volunteers would go into patients' homes, assess what was needed, and get it done. Soon, he was hosting a monthly informal support group for his volunteers. They talked openly about what the work entailed for them and what it cost them emotionally. In that setting, Kevin honed his knowledge of the moral dilemmas that caregivers must come to terms with, in order to survive their work.

He moved to England, earned a master's degree in bioethics, then moved home to care for his aging parents. Now he's combined every practical how-to he learned with every ethical quandary he's negotiated to come up with a guide that I believe may be a way to haul MAiD providers off the moral precipices from which we're bound to find ourselves dangling.

Knowing that there won't be simple right and wrong choices with track two MAiD requests—only hard options— Kevin created the IDEA rubric to formulate a last best judgment. Identify the facts. Determine the principles in conflict. Explore available options in clinical, legal, ethical, and organizational terms, using the social determinants of health. Act on the best option.

Why is the IDEA framework so helpful? Because it considers both the patient's request and the practitioner's distress in carrying out that request. It balances what we doctors ought to do against what we can. It acknowledges that when I insert myself into a patient's life—as I did with Thor and with Tom—I can tip them toward hope or toward despair.

Today Thor would have qualified as a track two patient, and his life would have been shortened by a year. His daughters would have missed all those weekends, all those walks in the sunshine. They also wouldn't have had to face his stroke, his fracture, and his hospitalization. Would they feel relief? Would they have missed the extra time? Questions that have no answers, I know.

Now when I ask a patient who is requesting MAiD, "Is there anything that could happen that would change your mind?" I ask it knowing the limits imposed by aging, social isolation, poverty, racialization, lack of education, uneven health care resources. I ask it so that together my patient and I can make our last best judgment. Not the right decision or the only one. But our best. That gives me some comfort. Will it be enough, going forward, to give long-term sufferers and the mentally ill a good end of life, a good death? We'll have to see.

In the end, a good death comes down to listening. Listening is an act of generosity. It's empathy. It's care.

It's hard to describe all the nuances I hear when a patient tells me their story, but what I'm alert for is suffering. Sometimes I can hear it in the first utterance. Sometimes I hear it in the anticipation of pain, or loss of purpose, or mind, or will to live. Knowing that I am alleviating someone's suffering is what makes this work doable. The story tells me the why and the why now, but it isn't all I need to hear. The whole story plumbs which resources they are getting and which they are not. Their doubts and questions. What details have been missed? What paths have gone unexplored? Who isn't listening?

Early on in this work, one of my mentors said trenchantly, "If the patient says they are suffering, it is not up to you to validate it. They are." And if the patient says that suffering is irremediable by any means available or acceptable to them, it is.

So when I hear the suffering, I assure the person of their eligibility—and then I listen harder. Because that's the moment they begin to ease up, to show me their true selves. I've *heard* them. They don't have to convince me of the "rightness" of their request. They can just talk to me. That is a moment of great comfort for both of us. That's where a good death begins.

I have been a journeyman in this work. I started out with the convictions forged during my years of practice, when I had to stand by helplessly while my patients suffered in silence and isolation, wanting a dignified end to their struggles. Often, because of the way our system of specialists is structured, I was shut out of their planning to secure that goal, or at least to end pain and dependence. When I did act, it was under the cover of relieving suffering, anticipating death as a welcome consequence. So much unspoken understanding with families, so much shared agony of action, without being able to acknowledge what we were really doing. I would never want to go back to those days.

That's why I embraced MAiD so wholeheartedly and embrace it still. But looking back on the early days, I'm nonplussed that I once took pride in being able to do a full assessment in sixty minutes. Now I've learned not to rush. I don't want to. I want to know these people, to understand their characters and what has shaped them. Our conversation weaves back and forth from their parents to their children, the threads that have woven the quilt of their lives. And it is a quilt—old patches and new ones, dark periods interspersed with happy memories, hardships faded and softened with time, triumphs now cherished and warm in the telling.

Believe me, it can be tough. We are parsing the value of a life. Is being aware of the month, the weather, of food and taste enough to wake up for every day? Do we act now to avoid what we fear the most—the loss of our memories, our increasing frailty, our decreasing independence? Do we hope for more time, or do we release hope like a balloon and find comfort in watching it drift away on the wind?

Deciding there is no longer enough reason to persist in living is intricate. It may free a person of obligations to others. They now act for themselves alone. Their needs move to the forefront. But by this very move, the sensibilities of family and caregivers take a back seat. It can feel selfish. We have to acknowledge that. There is always a cost to ending a life.

The journey we go on with these patients matters. They want choice and they want control. Their dignity is wrapped up in the values they espouse about purpose, honour, and suffering. And grace. After nearly fifty years of trying to battle illness and death, I stand in awe of their choice. After a lifetime of priding myself on my independence, I find myself strangely satisfied and humbled to join forces with palliative care teams, specialists, and care providers, and to realize I am no longer going it alone.

As I listen to my patients and fellow care providers, I hear my own words differently. I hear caring, I hear frustration, and I sometimes hear despair. But my greatest comfort is when I hear serenity. When I know I can give them the dignity and respect and peace they seek. That is a comfort, too.

The Way Ahead

MAiD is changing as you read this. The delivery of MAiD is shifting quickly and in major ways that will answer many of the concerns that plagued me in my early years of provisions. These changes also will help the many Canadians who find the rules around qualifying for MAiD too restrictive. And yes, they will raise new concerns that will require new ways of thinking and working together.

At the Legislative Level

Because Canada's legislators passed Bill C-7 in March 2021, Canadians whose natural death isn't yet reasonably foreseeable are able to request assisted dying. Until that point, MAiD doctors like me were applying the RFND clause broadly. That allowed me to provide for a patient like Ashley, who had an incredibly rare neurodegenerative condition, even though she was only twenty-eight. Under this new legislation, the door opened for patients like Thor, Tom, and so many others to ask for help to die on their own terms, earlier than I was able to provide for them. My obligation to explore all means to relieve their suffering still stands, but what I learned about them and their values has shifted how I will proceed in the future.

Initially, I feared the increased workload that servicing track two patients would require. Dr. Andrea Frolic's prediction regarding our limited human resources haunted me a little bit. But as it has turned out, every MAiD case seems to require some extra effort. Glitches happen no matter how many times you run the checklist. Nurses may not arrive to put in IV lines—sorry again, Yolanda—or a relative's late request to attend makes us shift our schedule. MAiD is never routine, nor should it be.

The new amendments have increased our obligations as MAiD providers. I'm going to quote the law here to show you how extensively. We must review the available means of "counselling services, mental health and disability support services, community services, and palliative care." In addition, the person seeking MAiD must also be "offered consultations with relevant professionals who provide those services." Finally, the person and physicians or nurse practitioners must discuss "the reasonable and available means to relieve the person's suffering and . . . agree with the person that the person has given them serious consideration."

As I've noted, that phrase "available means" is fraught. It underscores the scarcity of these resources, especially in rural and remote areas. Available services may be fractured among different tiers of government or trapped in silos that fail to address the specific needs of disadvantaged populations, such as inner-city unhoused people and displaced Indigenous Peoples.

Working with track two patients whose deaths aren't reasonably foreseeable requires professionals beyond physicians; nurse practitioners, physiatrists, social workers, psychiatrists, counsellors, religious professionals, and volunteers. Some institutions are already working to provide a pool of experts who can offer the clinical expertise a MAiD provider needs to validate a patient's request. I don't hesitate to reach out to these experts; I'm grateful to have their measured, comprehensive response and am relieved if they step up to offer something beyond the stark life-or-death choices our patients are obliged to consider. CAMAP, true to its mission, remains a vital source of information, mutual support, and encouragement as we MAiD practitioners shoulder this new burden in our practices.

When the pandemic exposed the disgraceful state of our long-term care facilities, Canadians loudly demanded that provincial governments raise the standards or offer other places to age and die with dignity. What also became clear is just how vital human connection is, and how caring for each other and taking responsibility for our most frail citizens define who we as Canadians want to be.

As we practitioners continue to hone our skills in providing MAiD to relieve our patients' suffering, we're more aware than ever of the need to affirm the value of a life, the dignity inherent in it, and the rightness of having a choice. But only if we are already assured that the fundamentals of respectful caring are in place.

Here's how I now assess patients with Alzheimer's disease for MAiD. I recognize that it is a terminal condition with an average trajectory of six to ten years from diagnosis to death; this allows me to reassure patients concerning their eligibility. I watch their condition closely, checking in every three or four months. When I sense that their capability to understand their request for MAiD is becoming critically low, I signal my concern and we set a date.

Why? Because I practice in Ontario, where patients must be able to consent *in the moment*.

Currently, federal law allows for a final consent waiver: a patient can come to an agreement with their MAiD provider that an assisted death will be provided on or before a set date if they have lost capacity before that date. However, these waivers can only be written up *after* the person has met the eligibility criteria for MAiD as a track one patient.

Quebec, however, has been leading the way to more inclusive options. In 2015, the province's government brought into force the Act Respecting End-of-Life Care. This act enfolded assisted dying into the broad obligations of end-of-life services for Quebecers. Quebec surged ahead again in 2019, when the Superior Court of Québec ruled RFND to be unconstitutional. That motivated Canada's Parliament to fall in line and harmonize the law through Bill C-7.

And I was heartened that in June 2023, quietly and without fanfare, the Quebec legislature passed into law Bill 11, which made advance requests legal in that province. Such an advance request, or AR, is made *before* the person meets all of the eligibility criteria for MAiD and allows that person to have an assisted death once they do meet the criteria, even if that time comes after they lose decision-making capacity.

The vast majority of Canadians already support allowing people to make advance requests for MAiD. They want legalized advance requests that permit them to have an assisted death even if they have lost their capacity to consent on the day. Such requests would acknowledge our aging population, and help assuage the dread that many of us feel about being warehoused in long-term care facilities, unable to engage with our community or recognize our loved ones. The isolation imposed during the 2020 COVID lockdown starkly underscored that fear. We doctors hear it all the time: "Don't let me end up in a nursing home, a shell of myself, not knowing my family." The AR is intended to bring peace of mind and to allay that dread.

Imagine what the option of an advance request would mean for someone who has received a diagnosis of a serious and incurable illness such as Alzheimer's disease. They could, with their loved ones' blessing, put in place arrangements to ensure their assisted death, once they met the circumstances that they themselves had defined as intolerable. Even if they were robbed of decision-making capacity on the day, those closest to them would know that they are following carefully considered wishes and plans.

Naturally, Quebec put safeguards in place when they passed Bill 11 that will be enacted over the next two years. At the time of the AR, a patient must have the capacity to understand that request and its consequences; they must have a diagnosis that anticipates their losing the capacity to consent; and they must anticipate that their assisted death will occur after they lose that capacity.

The eligibility criteria remain largely the same, with one addition. The person in question still must have a serious disease, illness, or disability; be in an advanced state of irreversible decline in capability; and be experiencing unbearable physical or psychological suffering that cannot be relieved under conditions they find acceptable. The new requirement is that before the patient can be helped to die, two independent assessors must agree that they see *observable* signs of enduring physical and psychological suffering that match those set forth in the AR.

Here's how it will work: a doctor or nurse practitioner will have made an initial diagnosis and outlined the expected course of the illness with the patient. They may then help the patient to itemize clearly what behaviours or physical signs will indicate "observable suffering" when the time comes that the patient cannot do this for themselves. Future MAiD assessors, even if they come into the picture years later, must be sure that the observable suffering documented in the directive arises from the patient's diagnosis and their understanding of the course of their disease. These assessors will also discuss the request with the members of the patient's regular care team and loved ones.

There's more: the patient must understand when they are making the AR that MAiD still might not occur. Even if the suffering appears to be arising from the diagnosis, the two assessors must agree that objectively, the suffering is enduring, unbearable, and irremediable, and that all other eligibility criteria have been met.

The patient may—and probably should—involve in their AR a trusted third party, whose role is to signal to caregivers that the time has come to put the request in play. Patients can also add a trusted fourth party, in case the third party is not available, or refuses or neglects to initiate the request.

The document is signed and dated by the patient, the doctor or nurse practitioner who has been guiding the conversation, and the trusted third (and, perhaps, fourth) party. This signing happens in the presence of a notary, or in the presence of two witnesses who also sign and affirm that the document contains the advance request of the patient. Then the document is recorded in a to-be-established registry or with the officiating notary.

The patient may withdraw their request or replace it with a new one, as long as they have the capacity to do so. Finally, when the trusted party/parties recognize that the time has come, they will call in two independent assessors, who will confirm that the stated criteria have been observed and then approve the MAiD provision.

How might this look for a practitioner such as myself if Canada follows Quebec's lead in 2024? Let's imagine a senior living at home with Alzheimer's, at a moderate stage of decline. They may have a spouse, perhaps aging or unwell themselves, as a primary, 24/7 caregiver; they may have children, friends, PSWs, or other visitors who take on some of the care and companionship needs.

My own mother, in her decline, attended a senior's day program, where she socialized and participated in various activities. But she hated going, because she was so anxious on the van ride there. Were we increasing her misery by forcing her out of her cocoon? Maybe. But when she was at home alone, her anxiety often would drive her to call the police. "You have to do something about your mother," a constable told my sister.

The grim reality is that cognitive decline is so slow that our loved ones are often in crisis before we realize how bad it's become. Or there is an event—most often a fall—that lands them in hospital, and it becomes clear that more care will be needed in future than can be provided at home.

Let's assume that our hypothetical patient with Alzheimer's and his family realize that such a future is coming and that he decides to set up an advance request with me. I make sure to discuss the prognosis of Alzheimer's disease with him and his wife. He is adamant that he already knows what it is and how it looks (perhaps he has seen his own parent suffer the disease), but I explain that the moderate stages of the disease can last for many years, and we will use cognitive tools to measure its progress going forward.

I suggest he prepare a document that clearly states the specific observable behaviours and needs, arising out of his illness, that would signal grievous and unbearable suffering for him.

He and his wife prepare his list and we review it at length. They decide that when he needs help dressing and toileting; when he requires constant supervision; when his ability to use and understand language has substantially diminished; when his mood varies between placid and volatile; when his interest in the broader world has significantly diminished and he has lost life-long skills such as piano playing; and when he misidentifies his wife and children more often than not—these are the observable behaviours and needs that would trigger the implementation of his request for an assisted death without consent in the moment.

The patient designates his wife to be his trusted third party, and we discuss whether he wants one of his children to be a trusted fourth party. We sign and date his request and convene two witnesses to attest that the document contains the patient's Advance Request, and they sign and date it as well. Then I file the document with his other key medical information, and also submit it to the yet-to-be created registry and to the patient's lawyer.

And if the patient's general situation remains fairly stable while his condition declines, then we can hope the process of triggering his AR will go smoothly. But let us imagine that it is several years in the future; I have retired, and his wife died suddenly not long after they filed the AR. The patient's children have moved him to a long-term care facility with a memory ward. Though the patient seems content there, he's becoming increasingly passive, speaking very little, able to eat only soft mush, and regularly unable to recognize his family members. His son—whom the patient added as a trusted third party in an amendment to the original request after the death of his wife—asks his father's lawyer for the

AR. He wants to be sure that his father is not suffering in the ways that he had expressly designated as unbearable to him.

If the son decides that his father has indeed slipped into the state that he had dreaded, the process now passes to his care facility. Two assessors must agree that the patient's behaviour and needs, as observed by them, is evidence of enduring and intolerable suffering based on his prior expressed criteria.

The next step is not necessarily a simple one, however. In territories that have permitted advance requests, heated debates have arisen with regard to the law, to ethics, to the medical community's duty of care, and to our collective values. It is not and never will be a straightforward path. Yet it is an option that most aging Canadians want, even though the vast majority will never request MAiD. The bigger challenge, even thornier and more pressing, is providing our elders a true alternative: dignified, holistic, respectful, and safe homeplaces to end their days when their own home is not a possibility. Such facilities exist—at a high price. To make them more available, more Canadians will have to band together to demand them from our governments, and follow through on those demands.

If advance directives are a hot-button issue, Mental Disorders as the Sole Underlying Medical Condition (MD-SUMC) to request MAiD is a potential conflagration. It is so divisive and enmeshed with societal, historical, and clinical beliefs and assumptions that the Quebec Assembly specifically excluded mental disorder as a criterion in Bill 11.

Fifty years after the introduction of antipsychotic medications, which allowed formerly institutionalized patients to rejoin their communities, we are still questioning both our understanding of mental disorders and effective treatments for them.

Yet people suffering from mental disorders deserve the same rights as every other Canadian. Even if their diagnoses shift over time, should their suffering be considered of a different order because it stems from a mental disorder rather than a physical or neurological one?

"Irreversible" is a key point of contention. It is true that some sufferers from mental disorders improve or recover without any treatment at all, or in response to a particular treatment after others have been tried and failed. Thus how can a mental disorder ever be certain to meet the eligibility criteria of *irreversible* illness? How can we be precise in assessing a patient who is seeking MAiD for unremitting depression?

What I know for certain is that many of my patients with chronic and debilitating conditions have attempted suicide, and many more despair about the state of their life to the point of suicidal ideation. Often patients who request MAiD don't share these kinds of thoughts with me until I assure them they're eligible—then the floodgates open. They share how deeply they've been suffering, and express relief that it will end on their terms, with their core values intact.

So how do we distinguish between a patient's suicidal ideation and a genuine desire for MAiD? Determining suicidality is a part of every assessment I make. As the legislation moves forward, a patient's care team will really need to step up. We will need to consider all of the patient's treatments over time, the successes and the failures. It will not be a quick process.

As I write this in October 2023, MD-SUMC is due to come into effect nationally in March 2024. A training curriculum for MAiD assessors and providers, developed by CAMAP and rendered through Queens University, is up and running across Canada. It will ensure consistency in approach and deliver the highest standards of clinical care and support for us all, patients and practitioners alike.

This will be a difficult journey, and MAiD providers will require the support of each patient's care team. None of us can afford to be confrontational or territorial; we must be inclusive. We must explore all other possible approaches to relieving a patient's suffering, but can never lose sight of the person who is requesting assistance to die on their own terms.

At the Local Level

When COVID-19 shut down our lives as we knew them, MAiD providers, like everyone else, adapted to virtual platforms. As a result, the geographic range of whom I could assess expanded; my face entered homes hundreds of kilometres away via screens. Families around the globe joined in on my Zoom visits with their elders. In many ways, the connection was easier and richer.

Online MAiD assessments worked in a pinch, but actual provisions were a different story, as I described with my long-time patient Gayle. Constrained by limited contact, masked, goggled, and gloved, I felt like I was making a hazardous services call, rather than providing a good death. We had limited time to express our respect and gratitude, to reflect on the life lived. Few were permitted to say farewell in person, and goodbyes felt diminished on screen. Touch became tentative and rare.

But as life returns to normal, I will continue to employ virtual platforms in my MAiD practice. Nothing replaces face-to-face contact, but I can save time and energy; I can see more patients; and more family members can check in and be seen, not just heard. As a by-product, I've loved watching seniors become nimble with technology such as iPads and video calls. What had been a reach in providing for Ashley is now routine.

Another area that's improving is the connection between MAiD services and funeral homes. In a MAiD provision, every patient has their own hopes for location, comfort, and space. Some people love the separate rooms that hospitals and institutions have created for MAiD. (I still smile at the memory of Joe's provision at Scarborough Grace.) Others, like Yolanda, find them impersonal. As numbers rise for patients seeking assisted deaths, I hope funeral homes continue to adapt, to be ready to assist families wherever a MAiD provision occurs, and to make the transition to their locations smooth, anxiety-free, and welcoming.

Here's a change I find hopeful. The Office of the Chief Coroner in Ontario now asks providers to verify if the patient identifies as disabled (that took some exploration in terminology), Indigenous (First Nations, Inuit, Metis), and/ or belonging to any ethnic/racial group. Gender identification has broadened. MAiD providers ask our patients if they feel marginalized, disadvantaged, or live in poverty; we document which disability services are provided and the length of time they have been in effect.

The goal of this Canada-wide documentation is to identify gaps in services and to offer better care to our disadvantaged, marginalized, and racialized populations. In this way, MAiD reporting is part of a cultural groundswell, as all Canadians learn a greater respect for Indigenous Peoples and acknowledge how our most marginalized have been neglected. But this documentation must be followed by action, to redistribute resources so that every Canadian lives the best life they can. We are a big country with a small population, but this is one way we could lead the world.

I'd also like to make one last plea to family doctors to consider adding MAiD provisions as an extension of the care you offer patients. Initially, those of us who did MAiD had to be self-taught, because there were no programs. We had to become experts, because we were developing standards of practice to balance legislative restraints with our patients' pleas to relieve their suffering. Now much of that work has been done; we don't need to be a subspecialty. In 2023 CAMAP will launch a nation-wide curriculum developed for practitioners by MAiD experts representing diverse locations and disciplines. In the meantime, CAMAP offers mentorship and sympathetic consultation to all its members and, it can't be said too often, heartfelt support in the tough times. As new legislation expands eligibility criteria, doctors will run into more and more complex issues with patients who request assisted death. I already hear it, as I discuss these issues with my colleagues. They are a grand, thoughtful, caring, sharing bunch. It fills me with pride to be among them. But we can't do it alone—we will need all hands on deck.

As I've mentioned, most of my MAiD patients were referred to me—word spreads, other doctors refer, families call, Julie Campbell sends request my way from the ministry's MAiD site. In my first five years, only three of the people I provided came from my family practice, Irene being the first. Providing MAiD is never going to be routine, but if all family doctors did it, no one would have to do so many.

During the past few years I have spent far more time than before online; my notion of life-long learning has exploded, and necessarily so. Advancements in molecular biology, genetic tailoring, robotic engineering, and AI technology have led to new treatments and cures. I follow progress in the treatment for such conditions as Parkinson's, multiple sclerosis, ALS, and dementia that would have been unheard of even ten years ago. I am diligent in flagging new understandings around depression, PTSD, and many other mental health challenges. Just-in-time learning has been at the core of my work and will be a necessary boon for all who come after.

Younger colleagues who are just entering the world of patient care will have tools to alleviate or slow patient decline in ways I can't begin to imagine. But even so armed, they will still need to truly hear and understand their patient's suffering when the requests come. In an aging society, longevity without quality of life is the driver of many requests for Medical Assistance in Dying. It is why MAiD was initially legalized, why I became a MAiD doctor, and why we must all work hard to ensure longevity *with* quality of life.

At the same time, I accept that providing MAiD is a unique service, and I accept its unique burdens. Doctors do not want to kill their patients. My concept of cradle-to-grave care may be outdated—seniors live longer, doctors retire, care is siloed, families move. The result is a detached kindness in practising MAiD, and maybe that's not such a bad thing, for either doctor or patient.

But even if most family doctors won't come aboard—in seven years, I think I've managed to recruit three—others will. Nurse practitioners, who undertake their responsibilities with conviction and passion. Palliative care doctors, who transition their patients when the time is right. I see their intense commitment in action, confident and sure that we can embrace this expanding challenge. Our numbers may never be large, so it is essential for us to support each other in this invaluable service we provide to Canadians.

An end to intolerable suffering. A dignified, peaceful exit, honouring the patient, their values, and the meaning of their lives. A moment of grace. We all want that. I'm honoured to help provide it.

ACKNOWLEDGEMENTS

Supreme Court decisions have far-reaching effects on the lives of citizens. But the unanimous nine-to-zero ruling in 2015, which amended the criminal law to allow Canadians medical assistance to die, had an instant effect on me.

It shifted the direction of my medical practice; and it affirmed my life-long belief that ensuring a dignified death without suffering is what we all want for our patients. I could now put my beliefs into practice.

This book would not have been written if I hadn't met and walked with Yolanda Martins through her own battle with cancer in the aftermath of her lung transplant. Her urgent imperative to have a dignified death fuelled this project. Yolanda was unlike many of my patients: she'd spent her professional life in the field of initiating and analyzing studies related to quality of life and death issues around cancer treatment and palliative care.

My co-author, Johanna Schneller, came aboard early. This was crucial to moving this book away from the privacy constraints of patient confidentiality and bringing it into the public eye. Without her initial interview of Yolanda, I could not have conceived the unique collaboration that resulted in our being able to tell other patient stories that are at the centre of the MAiD experience. She and I have reached out to the families of the patients whose stories are told here so that I could name them. Our motive was to respect their lives and to frame their unique contribution in helping us and our readers understand their journey in assisted dying. Offering their permission is an act of courage on their part, and we are both deeply grateful for their time, openness, and generosity. I hope Johanna and I have been able to justly honour the memory of those they have loved.

The writing of this book has also underscored what I have learned about my convictions, frailties, and passion about dying bravely.

Many mentors and teachers came to my aid as I undertook this journey from simply wanting to provide MAiD to knowing how to do so. As I pursued my often-murky goals, Dr. Jeff Myers sling-shot me into the world of palliative care and landed me in settings I could not have imagined without his confidence in me and his unfailing support. There were no MAiD doctors in Canada, so there was no precedent for learning how to be a MAiD doctor.

My undying regard also extends to the many other doctors who shepherded me along the way: Arnell Baguio, Sandra Black, Sandy Buchman, Andrea Frolic, David Kendal, Denise Marshall, and Kevin Real. There are many more MAiD doctors whose personal stories have always resonated with me. I know that our goals are shared in this serious business but sometimes a dollop of dark humour never fails to lighten the load of duty and care.

Doctors cannot do this work without the support of the nurses, care coordinators, and pharmacists who are the foundations for the service we provide. A hearty thanks to nurse practitioner Julie Campbell, who has filled many hours of road trips discussing thorny issues and possible solutions. And to my strong right arm, Yuri Zachariah, the go-to nurse who saved the day with Yolanda and has never failed to answer my sometimes-panicked calls for help with instant and unstinting aid.

The growth of MAiD across Canada would also have been a ragged affair if it weren't for the creation of CAMAP. The Canadian Association of Medical Assessors and providers is the MAiD providers' online grassroots organization that provides support, comradeship, and professional learning for assessors and providers alike. Its early formation in 2016 and strong organization led to it becoming a beacon for the legislative changes reflected in Bill C-7, which advances the original MAID legislation. CAMAP will remain invaluable in all that is yet to come for Canadians around medically assisted death.

Johanna and I have been encouraged from the start by our publisher Penguin Canada. They have provided unfailing support and editorial expertise throughout the entire process—especially Diane Turbide in the early days and her successor Lara Hinchberger, who came aboard in 2021 and enabled us to hone the essential heart of the narrative. Our thanks also go to Amy Moore-Benson and Michael Levine, our agents, who have come together to support each of their authors in unison.

I owe my husband Bob Ramsay my eternal gratitude. Bob writes every day, and it is the heart of his values and belief, so he is the model of what it takes. He has always been my first and well-meant harshest critic. Reframing what he calls "physician-speak" is no mean feat, and I have emerged, I hope, with a clearer and more personal account. It certainly has not come willingly or easily.

My children have never wavered in their support of my determination to be a MAiD doctor, and to write about it. My youngest, listening to an urgent call I took on a Saturday as we were driving home from a shopping trip, commented, "Well, at least all these calls make sense to me now. They need you."

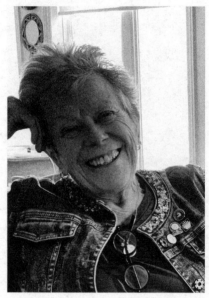

© Bob Ramsay

JEAN MARMOREO is a doctor, writer, advocate, athlete, and adventurer. She is a specialist in end-of-life medicine and was one of the first doctors in Canada to provide MAiD—Medical Assistance in Dying—when it became legal in 2016. Jean was a regular columnist for *The Globe and Mail* and the *National Post,* and is the author of *The New Middle Ages: Women in Midlife.*

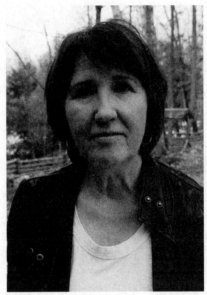

© Johanna Schneller

JOHANNA SCHNELLER is one of North America's leading freelance journalists, specializing in entertainment features. Her cover stories have appeared in *Vanity Fair*, *InStyle*, *Premiere*, *More*, and *Ladies' Home Journal*. Johanna co-wrote the bestselling books *Uncontrollable* with Mark Towhey and *Woman Enough* with Kristen Worley.